D0586001

THE HISTORY OF MEDICINE SERIES

ISSUED UNDER THE AUSPICES

OF THE LIBRARY OF THE

NEW YORK ACADEMY OF MEDICINE

———————

No. 36

LIBRARY PUBLICATIONS COMMITTEE

NEW YORK ACADEMY OF MEDICINE

William B. Ober, M.D., *Chairman*

Gertrude L. Annan	Saul Jarcho, M.D.
Paul F. Cranefield, M.D., Ph.D.	Samuel W. Lambert, Jr., M.D.
James E. McCormack, M.D.	William D. Sharpe, M.D.

THE CITY THAT WAS

by
STEPHEN SMITH

138135

and
*The Report of the
General Committee of Health,
New York City, 1806*

With a preface by
JOHN DUFFY

Published under the auspices of the Library of
The New York Academy of Medicine

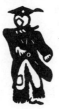

RA448
N5 S57
1973

Scarecrow Reprint Corporation
Metuchen, N. J.   1973

The City That Was was originally published by Frank Allaben, New York, 1911, and is reprinted 1973, including a new preface and the 1806 *Report of the General Committee of Health,* N.Y.C.

All materials used in preparing this reprint are from the collection of the Library of The New York Academy of Medicine.

Library of Congress Cataloging in Publication Data

Smith, Stephen, 1823-1922.
    The city that was.

    (The History of medicine series)
    "Published under the auspices of the Library of
the New York Academy of Medicine."
    Reprint of 2 works published separately in 1911
and 1806, respectively. The second work was pub-
lished as part of Documents relating to the Board
of Health.
    Includes bibliographical references.
    1. Hygiene, Public--New York (City).
2. Sanitation. I. New York (City). General
Committee of Health. The report of the General
Committee of Health, New York City, 1806. 1972.
II. Title. III. Title: The report of the
General Committee of Health, New York City. 1806.
IV. Series.
RA448.N5S57 1973   614'.09747'1   73-1827
ISBN 0-8108-0598-7

Copyright 1973
The New York Academy of Medicine

EDITORS' NOTE

The old charge of the ivory tower has been leveled in recent years against established academia. This includes not only academic medicine but historians in general and historians of medicine. The current cry is for "relevance." To meet this challenge we have republished Stephen Smith's *The City That Was,* a book written in 1911 when its author had retired and could look backward with a perspective of half a century upon the reforms in public health and sanitation which he had helped initiate. To this we have appended the brief *Report of the General Committee of Health* for 1806.

The slums are not a new invention, nor is their character altered by calling them a ghetto; euphemisms may serve the purposes of polemicists, but they are out of place in the field of public health.

The city fathers of 1806 and 1866 had to face the problems created by an influx of immigrants who were poor, ill-fed, ill-clothed, ill-housed. They were crowded into wretched hovels perched on an accumulation of human waste, correctly labeled "fever nests." Basic facilities, let alone amenities for maintenance of minimal decency and cleanliness were lacking. There were not enough doctors to treat the sick, and the rate of illness among the poor was higher than that of the more financially stable population. Unlike rural poverty, which is widely spaced and less conspicuous, urban poverty is — and was — highly visible.

The same problem exists in our urban slums today. Poverty, accompanied by its handmaidens, ignorance and fear, continues to threaten health and life; in a real sense it is the background for much of human disease. We may no longer have epidemics of smallpox, cholera, and typhoid as in the nineteenth century, but these fevers have been replaced by other diseases, those suitable for the civilized twentieth century.

However, progress was made, and today we reap the benefit. No longer do visitors to New York City have to fear that they will carry smallpox back to their families. No longer does a dinner guest contract typhoid fever from eating oysters in the restaurants of New York, but he does run the risk of viral hepatitis. Consumption no longer gallops, but the highest incidence of tuberculosis continues to be found among slum dwellers. There is still room for more progress.

In an article celebrating the 100th anniversary of New York City's Board of Health, Leona Baumgartner outlined the events of the 1860's:

> As pressures for reform mounted in New York City, the new health laws of England were studied. A private organization, the New York Association for Improving the Conditions of the Poor, later merged with the Charity Organization Society, today called the Community Service Society. Soon a number of influential persons in the city became alarmed. Peter Cooper, the merchant-prince-philanthropist, William Cullen Bryant, poet and editor of the *New York Evening Post*, Stephen Smith, and Norman B. Eaton, a lawyer, took over the task of collecting the facts on sanitary conditions in the tenement house district. Reform was demanded. The New York Academy of Medicine put pressure on the legislature. Smith's appeals to the legislature were in vivid, lurid, and human terms. One legislator cried, 'Why, I believe I have got smallpox, for I begin to itch all over,' as he heard a description of how wholesale dealers sold clothing manufactured in homes where the clothes had covered the beds of children with smallpox and remembered that he had just bought a suit from one of these dealers.
>
> The reformers were helped by the threat of a new epidemic of cholera. Finally, they overcame the long-standing opposition of a corrupt alliance of Tammany Democrats and upstate Republicans, whose legislation had failed to handle effectively

the growing threats to the health of the people in the city. A new administrative structure was set up by the state legislature in 1866 as part of an effort to achieve reform in all phases of municipal government.*

The confrontation of today is with *The City That Is*. It is only by examining the problems of the past, analyzing the steps taken to solve them, and reviewing the results, that an informed approach can be made to the problems of today. And it has become a cliché to quote the aphorism, "Those who do not learn the lesson of history are doomed to repeat it."

G.L.A.
W.B.O.

---

*Baumgartner, Leona, "ONE HUNDRED YEARS OF HEALTH: New York City, 1866-1966," *Bulletin of the New York Academy of Medicine,* Second Series, v.45, #6, pp.555-586, June 1969.

THE CHOLERA AND FEVER NESTS OF NEW YORK CITY.

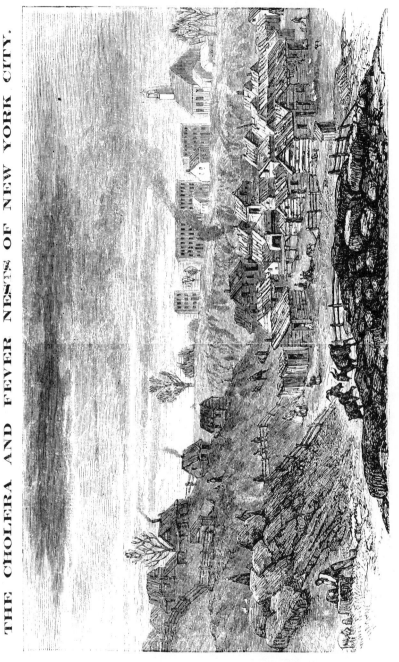

SHANTIES ON EIGHTH AVENUE.

PREFACE
To the 1973 Reprint

In *The City That Was* Dr. Stephen Smith (1823-1922) depicts New York City in the days prior to the great sanitary revolution. During the decades of the 1850's and 1860's New York was experiencing all the worst aspects of industrialism and urbanism and few of the beneficial ones. The city's expanding population constantly exceeded available housing, with the result that the poor were packed ever tighter and tighter into the older dilapidated sections. The Croton water system was supplying relatively good water, but little of it was available to the slum dwellers. Often five to ten families shared one hydrant. The sewer system was designed primarily to take care of surface drainage, although the well-to-do were beginning to connect their water closets to it. In the slums crude overflowing privies were common, and frequently one or two privies served ten or more families.

Under these conditions sicknesses of all types were rampant and life was short. By this date, however, the appalling misery in which the great mass of poor lived was becoming all too evident, and there was a rising social consciousness among many middle and upper class citizens. In the United States the medical profession played an important role in drawing public attention to the deplorable health and environmental conditions. The author of *The City That Was*, Dr. Stephen Smith, was only one of a number of able, intelligent, and humane physicians who helped lead the drive for social and sanitary reforms. Long before Smith appeared on the scene, men such as Drs. John H. Griscom, Elisha Harris, and Joseph M. Smith, working through the New York Academy of Medicine and aided by civic leaders and newspaper editors, had been fighting to remedy the worst social abuses. The groundswell for reform was already gathering in the 1850's; Dr. Stephen Smith and his colleagues took advantage of its momentum and brought the New York City Health Department into existence.

Dr. Smith came from a small farm in upstate New York in 1850 to study medicine at the College of Physicians and Surgeons of Columbia University. Upon graduation he spent two years as a resident at Bellevue Hospital; here he first encountered the misery and degradation of the poor. The correlation between environmental conditions and disease was brought home to Smith when his curiosity was aroused on discovering that almost one hundred cases of typhus had come from a single tenement. On visiting it, he was appalled at the crowding and incredible filth. This experience led him to join the Citizens' Association, a civic reform group, and to become a key member of its "Council of Hygiene."

Ironically, the reformers were fighting a corrupt municipal government which held power by manipulating the illiterate poor who were the chief victims of the social and political system. To awaken the conscience of the middle and upper classes, in 1864 the Council of Hygiene undertook a sanitary survey of the city, designed to expose the filth and degradation of the fetid slums. The leading spirit of the Council was Dr. Elisha Harris, but he was so deeply involved in the work of the United States Sanitary Commission, a civilian group organized to bolster the inadequate medical services of the Union Army, that much of the work of the sanitary survey fell on the shoulders of Dr. Smith. Although Dr. Harris edited the final report, Dr. Smith was called upon to present its findings before the State Legislature in February 1865.[*]

By this date the demand for reform was coming from

---

[*] *The Sanitary Condition of the City:* Report of the Council of Hygiene and Public Health of the Citizens' Association of New York, 1866. (Reprinted 1972 by the Arno Press, New York, N.Y.)

many sources, but there is little doubt that results of the sanitary survey, which were given widespread publicity in the newspapers and journals, provided the final impetus to push the health reform bill for New York City through the State Legislature. After years of fighting for health reform, its proponents despaired of achieving success at the local level and by-passed the municipal government. They created a Metropolitan Board of Health, which was a State agency. It is paradoxical that Americans pay lipservice to local government but invariably turn to the State or Federal authorities when faced with major problems.

The passage of the Metropolitan Board of Health Act in 1866 was only the beginning of Dr. Smith's long and productive career. He was one of the Health Commissioners for the city from 1868 to 1875, played an important role as a founder and first president of the American Public Health Association, and served as a member of the short-lived National Board of Health. In collaboration with Dr. Elisha Harris, Smith also took leadership in establishing a State Board of Health for New York in 1880. His national reputation in the health field was recognized by President Cleveland, who named him as one of the three American delegates to the Ninth International Sanitary Conference held in Paris during 1894.

Over and above his role in the public health movement, Dr. Smith was an outstanding surgeon, an early American champion of antisepsis, the author of several surgical textbooks and of a host of papers. From 1853 to 1864 he was successively editor of the *New York Journal of Medicine* and the *American Medical Times*. In addition, he was Professor of Surgery and Anatomy in the Bellevue Hospital Medical College and was an active member of the Bellevue Hospital staff for fifty years.

When Dr. Smith published *The City That Was*, almost fifty years had elapsed since the passage of the Metropolitan Board of Health Act. During this period America had seen the sanitary movement sweep over the country and had witnessed the emergence of effective public health agencies at all levels of government. Public health was no longer the avocation of socially conscious citizens and physicians but a

ix

professional field within its own right. The vast changes brought about by the sanitary movement and its successor, the bacteriological revolution, had immensely changed American cities, and there were few New Yorkers who could recall what the city had been like in the days before the Civil War. Dr. Smith was ideally suited for writing *The City That Was*, since he had been acutely aware of social conditions and had played a major role in attempting to remedy them. He was eighty-eight when his book appeared, and he survived for another eleven years. To public health leaders in the early 20th century, Dr. Smith, whose life had spanned a century, symbolized the sanitary movement. It was little wonder that he became a legend in his own time. His pioneering work in medicine and public health guarantees him a place in history. *The City That Was* helps us to relive that history.

✻   ✻   ✻   ✻   ✻

The Report of the General Committee of Health carries us back to a time at the beginning of the 19th century when yellow fever was a major problem in New York City. The disease had first appeared in 1702, when it wiped out almost a tenth of the town's population, and had made occasional forays in the ensuing years, but it was not until the 1790's that it again reached major epidemic proportions. A series of outbreaks over an eleven-year period began in 1793. During this time three major epidemics occurred, one in 1793, when 750 residents died, another in 1798 with 1,524 deaths, and a third in 1803 causing 606 deaths. In the intervening years the annual summer death toll from the fever ranged from about 25 to 356. The final yellow fever attack in this period developed in the summer of 1805 and brought death to 262 New Yorkers. It was directly responsible for this report, which appeared in 1806.

Yellow fever is a horrible and highly fatal disorder. To New Yorkers, who knew nothing about pathogenic organisms and insect vectors, it was a strange, mysterious, and fearful pestilence. It struck indiscriminately among all age groups, and its incidence conformed to no rational pattern. Laymen generally assumed the pestilence to be a contagious one, imported from abroad, but most physicians had seen too many instances where the infection was confined to one member of a family and therefore favored an environmental theory. With some variations, this theory held that a combination of meteorological conditions joined with filth and crowding were responsible for creating a poisonous miasma which affected susceptible individuals. In the early days, when malaria, enteric disorders, and a host of other fever-producing diseases were endemic, summertime was considered the fever season. The miasmic theory maintained that a conjunction of the precise temperature and humidity with other environmental conditions could turn the customary summer fevers into a pestilential or malignant fever.

A major source of these pestilential fevers was thought to be putrefying substances such as human and animal wastes, garbage, offal, carrion, and so forth. Construction during the summer months which exposed the damp undersoil to the air or the draining of swamps and pools was also considered a dangerous source of miasma. This miasmatic thesis or environmentalist view of etiology was responsible for the sanitary reform movement of the later 19th century.

In response to the danger from epidemics of yellow fever, a voluntary health committee was first organized in New York City during 1793. Subsequently this body was given official status and it functioned quite effectively during the successive yellow fever outbreaks. Recognizing the value of its work, in January 1805 the City Council decided to expand the committee's authority and turn it into a Board of Health. This new Board performed yeoman work during the 1805 outbreak, and its members were reappointed the following December to serve during 1806. Seeking to prevent the recurrence of yellow fever, the Board promptly appointed a committee, headed by Alderman Wynant Van Zandt, Jr., to investigate all sources of infection and to find ways to eliminate the unsanitary conditions which were held at least in part responsible for the disease.

After consulting with local physicians and appealing to the public for suggestions, the committee submitted its report in January, 1806. The report emphasized the need for pure water and adequate drainage, and suggested that the "noxious exhalations" from graveyards could be a source of danger. In recommending the appointment of a "skillful engineer" and the planting of trees and shrubs, the committee anticipated the work of later reformers. More significant, the committee advocated a form of slum clearance when, noting that certain houses have "proved to be the principal seats of disease, and the graves of their tenants," it urged that they be turned into warehouses at public expense. Finally, like all public health bodies during these years, it avoided the issue of quarantine versus sanitation by concluding that a strict quarantine should be maintained during the yellow fever months. Although short, the report is of considerable interest, since its recommendations foreshadow the subsequent sanitary reform movement.

July, 1972   JOHN DUFFY
                              Mary Alden Burke Professor
                                 of History
                              University of Maryland

THE CITY THAT WAS

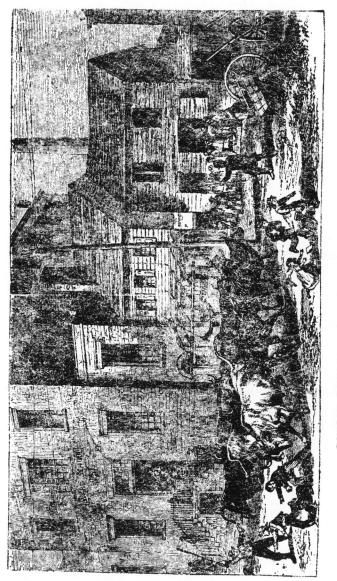

PUBLIC SCHOOL ADJOINING SLAUGHTER-PEN, 1865

THE CITY THAT WAS

By STEPHEN SMITH, A. M., M. D., LL. D.

COMMISSIONER OF THE METROPOLITAN BOARD OF HEALTH, 1868-1870;
COMMISSIONER OF THE BOARD OF HEALTH OF NEW YORK, 1870-1875

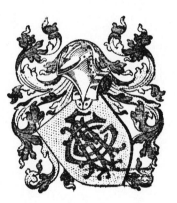

PUBLISHED BY FRANK ALLABEN
NUMBER THREE WEST FORTY-SECOND STREET, NEW YORK

COPYRIGHT, 1911, BY FRANK ALLABEN

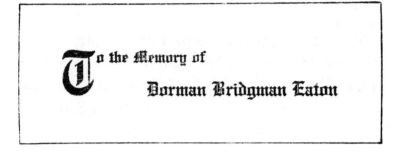

To the Memory of

Dorman Bridgman Eaton

My thanks are due especially to Mr. Frank Allaben and my son, Mr. Sidney Smith, for their service in carrying this book through the press.

STEPHEN SMITH.

NOTE BY THE PUBLISHER

THE story of a great life-saving social revolution, the mightiest in the nineteenth century and one of the most momentous in the nistory of civilization, is told here for the first time. It is told from the standpoint of the transformation of the City of New York, by a chief actor in the event.

Only by forcing ourselves into a receptive mood can we of the present credit the half of what is set before us concerning The City That Was. The shocked imagination rebels. It seeks relief in assuming that even a trained expert, a contemporaneous witness and investigator of the conditions described, in writing after they have passed away, unconsciously yields to the historian's temptation to throw the past into dramatic relief by starting exaggerations.

Dr. Smith, however, leaves us no room for doubt. The appalling chapter in which he lays bare the New York of 1864 is a contemporaneous document. It is a physician's report of a systematic medical inspection of New York in that year, as delivered before a Legislative Committee a few months later by the very physician who had directed the inspection.

Nevertheless, The City That Was is not New York alone. She is but a type. Her condition, with variations, may be multiplied, during the early years of the nineteenth century, by the total of the cities, towns, and villages in the world. In the work of regeneration some of these anticipated her. Others, including all throughout the territory of the United States, were aroused through her agitation and inspired by her example.

As a student of local history, the writer thought himself familiar with the many phases of the growth of New York; but the condition of the City as late as the period of our Civil War, as here depicted, startled him as might a revelation. He believes that no seriously minded man or woman can afford to ignore this volume. We owe it to ourselves and to one another fully to face its lesson. We shall be shocked; we shall be filled with horror; but accepting the city that now is, great as her faults may be, with a new gratitude, we shall turn with anointed sympathy and understanding to any earnest voice that pleads for the city that should be. And, indeed, other volumes which Dr. Smith himself has in preparation, as suggestive and as interesting as this one, may help us on in this direction.

FRANK ALLABEN

CONTENTS

I

A BLIND METROPOLIS AND HER DYING CHILDREN

II

A GREAT AWAKENING IN ENGLAND

III

THE AWAKENING IN AMERICA

IV

NEW YORK, THE UNCLEAN

V
VICTORY

VI

THE LEGAL WORK OF DORMAN BRIDGEMAN EATON

VII

THE OCCULT POWER OF FILTH

VIII

A CLOSING WORD

ILLUSTRATIONS

I

A Blind Metropolis and Her Dying Children

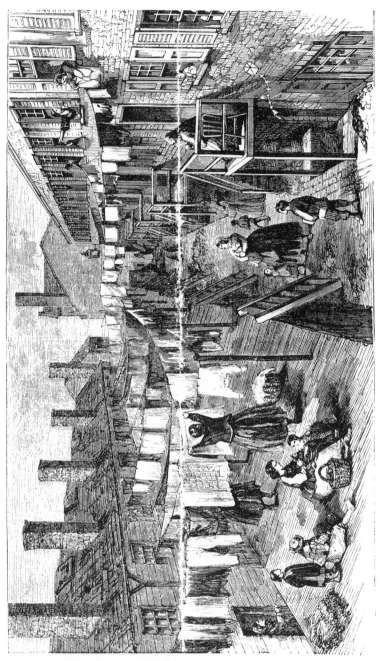

RIVAGION PLACE, GOERCK STREET.

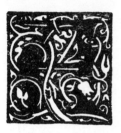GREAT problem was left for the first civilized inhabitants of New York to determine. Nature had made ample provision for the metropolis of the western hemisphere. But two possibilities were attached to its occupation by man — it could be healthy or unhealthy, at the option of the people.

THE conditions which made for health were: two large rivers of pure water, from the mountains and the sea, flushed its shores, carrying the outflow of its waste far away seaward; its soil could be thoroughly drained; its sewerage could be so constructed as to convey to the sea all forms of domestic waste and surface filth; its southern exposure towards the ocean insured sunlight and sea breezes; its inland situation supplied to its atmosphere the life-giving virtues of abundant vegetation; the climate was temperate.

Healthy or Unhealthy: Which?

The conditions which made for unhealthiness were: large areas of sodden marsh lands; a rock formation of shale, having a dip of the strata, nearly perpendicular, admitting the flow of surface water to great depths, thus poisoning springs and wells; numerous streams flowing into the rivers; large ponds of stagnant water; fierce summer heat.

FROM the year 1622 to the year 1866, a period of two hundred and forty-four years, the people elected that the city should be unhealthy. The land was practically undrained; the drinking water was from shallow wells, befouled by street, stable, privy, and other filth; there were no adequate sewers to remove the accumulating waste; the streets were the receptacles of garbage; offensive trades were located among the dwellings; the natural water courses and springs were obstructed in the construction of streets and dwellings, thus causing soakage of large areas of land, and stagnant pools of polluted water.

Two Centuries and a Half Unhealthy

Later, in these centuries of neglect of sanitary precautions, came the immigrants from every nation of the world, representing for the most part the poorest and most ignorant class of their respective nationalities. This influx of people led to the construction of the tenement house by landowners, whose aim was to build so as to incur the least possible expense and accommodate the greatest possible number. In dark, unventilated, uninhabitable structures these wretched, persecuted people were herded together, in cellars and garrets, as well as in the body of the building, until New York had the largest population to a square acre of any civilized city.

The people had not only chosen to conserve all the natural conditions unfavorable to health, but had steadily added unhygienic factors in their methods of developing the city.

THE result was inevitable. New York gradually became the natural home of every variety of contagious disease, and the favorite resort of foreign pestilences. Smallpox, scarlet fever, measles, diphtheria, were domestic pestilences with which the people were so familiar that they regarded them as necessary features of childhood. Malarial fevers, caused by the mosquitoes bred in the marshes, which were perfect culture-beds, were regularly announced in the autumnal months as having appeared with their "usual severity." The "White Plague," or consumption, was the common inheritance of the poor and rich alike.

A Plague-Stricken Town

With the immigrant, came typhus and typhoid fevers, which resistlessly swept through the tenement houses, decimating the poverty-stricken tenants. At intervals, the great oriental plague, Asiatic cholera, swooped down upon the city with fatal energy and gathered its enormous harvest of dead. Even "Yellow Fever," the great pestilence of the tropics, made occasional incursions and found a most congenial field for its operations.

F AILURE to improve the unhealthy conditions of the city, and the tendency to aggravate them by a large increase of the tenement-house population, offensive trades, accumulations of domestic waste, and the filth of streets, stables, and privy pits, then universal, caused an enormous sacrifice of life, especially among children. This fact is strikingly illustrated by the following comparison of figures taken from the official records.

Enormous Sacrifice of Life

The standard ratio of deaths to the total living in a community, where the death-rate is normal under proper sanitary conditions, has been fixed by competent authority at about 15 in 1,000 of population. The death-rate in New York, in the five years preceding 1866, averaged 38 in 1,000 population, which is 23 in excess of the normal standard of 15 in the 1,000. In a city with a population of 1,000,000, the estimated

population of New York in 1865, a death-rate
of 38 in the 1,000 means 23,000 deaths annually
from preventable diseases.

Mortality statistics computed on a scale of
forty years, the period during which New York
has been under an intelligent sanitary government, still more impressively show the former
waste of life through municipal neglect of the
elementary principles of public hygiene. The
lesson which these figures teach should be en-
graven on the memory of every man, woman,
and child. Our authority is the annual report
of the Department of Health of the City of New
York, for the year 1908, in which appears the
following statement.

"A remarkable decrease in the death-rate has
taken place within the past forty years, a decrease comparing each decennial rate with the
one immediately preceding represented by
seven, seven, and eighteen per cent respectively,
and comparing that of the first decennium with
the individual year under review, a decrease of
forty-seven per cent."

II

A Great Awakening in England

HOLERA was approaching the shores of England. The alarm of the people was intense. The enormous devastations of that pestilence on its first and only previous visit to that country, in 1832, were vividly recalled by the elder people. The only known preventive measures were "flight, fasting, and prayer." As the pestilence was believed to be a "visitation of God" on account of the sins of the people, the clergy petitioned the Prime Minister to proclaim a day of "fasting and prayer," with many expressions of sorrow at the prevailing national vices which had finally provoked the wrath of the Almighty. The Prime Minister replied in substance as follows:

The Scourge of 1849

"Do works meet for repentance. First make your homes and their surroundings clean and wholesome; then you may with propriety ask Almighty God to bless your efforts at protection against the approaching epidemic."

This response of the highest official of the

Kingdom to the usually humble and devout peti-
tion of the clergy, when the people were threat-
ened with an epidemic, was received with
profound astonishment by the religious classes,
with ridicule by the masses of the people, but
with commendation by sanitarians. The popular agitation was great. The clergy protested
with solemn asseverations their belief that pestilences were always indications that national
sins had become intolerable to the Almighty,
and only fastings and prayers could appease
His wrath.

The people at large gave no heed either to the
clergy's admonition to fast and pray, or to the
Prime Minister's advice to clean their homes
and their surroundings; but, with their usual
disregard of the domestic diseases with which
they were constantly familiar, gave no thought
to approaching danger. But the sanitarians
very earnestly urged the people of their respective localities to act upon the advice of the
Prime Minister, assuring them that cholera was
a disease which prevailed more generally and
severely in localities and homes where there
was the greatest amount of "filth."

The epidemic of 1849 came and went with its
apparent usual great disturbances of the people.
"Flight" and "fasting and prayers" had their
natural results, the former being effectual when
undertaken in time, and the latter without sensible influence over the mortuary records.

T HEN the net results of this visitation of
cholera were officially determined by
the Registrar General, one fact attracted
wide attention and created a profound and
lasting impression on the minds of the common
people. A town in the interior

Can Diseases
Be Prevented?
of England reported no case
of cholera, though the epidemic had prevailed with great
virulence in the communities surrounding it.

On inquiry as to the cause of this remarkable
feature of a pestilence that hitherto had shown
no respect for persons or localities, it was
learned that certain citizens of this town were
deeply impressed with the reasonableness of the
Prime Minister's suggestions, and had organized
and taken action accordingly. Volunteer committees composed of the leading men and women
were selected. One was to secure thorough
cleaning of the streets and public places; another was to cause an inspection of every residence and its surroundings and secure complete
cleanliness; a third was to obtain reports of all
cases of sickness and require immediate isola-
tion and treatment when there was the slightest
symptom of cholera.

This town had its "fastings and prayers," but
not until its citizens had done works meet for
repentance; and then it asked the divine bless-
ing on its efforts to protect itself — and its
prayers were abundantly answered.

But there was another phase of this place's experience not less impressive than its escape from cholera. There was a great diminution of such diseases as diphtheria, typhoid, erysipelas, scarlet fever, measles, and other low forms of sickness, so fatal in the homes of the poor, during the period that the citizens exercised so much care in securing cleanliness.

"A WORD fitly spoken is like apples of gold in pictures of silver." A word fitly spoken broke the spell of centuries, and completely revolutionized human history. That word was spoken, not at the suggestion of science, nor by a scientist, but, at the dictation of common sense, by a layman who happened to be in authority. It was a plain, simple word, which was understood by the people and which appealed to their common sense.

The Word Fitly Spoken

A new era now dawned upon the domestic life of the English people. Every household learned that cleanliness had not only saved a town from a visitation of cholera, but had reduced the contagious and infectious diseases always present in their homes. The Health Officer of England gave tremendous force to the revelation that had been made by officially characterizing and classifying cholera and the whole brood of domestic scourges as "filth diseases." This was a most happy term, because it suggested not only the source of these diseases, but the simple and effectual remedy that every householder could apply. It became popular in the sanitary literature of the period, and thus permeated all classes, until the most humble family knew its import and complied with its suggestion.

The next visitation of cholera to England was met by the simple remedy of domestic and civic cleanliness; and so manifestly effectual was this measure that the pestilence lost its former terrors. But the great and lasting gain to the people, which grew out of the original proclamation of the Prime Minister that cleanliness of the home and its surroundings was the best preventive of cholera, was the discovery of the fact that nearly all diseases which afflict the individual family, and in a larger sense the whole community, have their origin in or are intensified by decomposing waste matter, the "filth" of the sanitarian, in and around their homes.

So profoundly impressed with this fact were the laboring classes, and so earnest did they become in their zeal for sanitation, that sanitary measures entered into the political campaign. On one occasion a prominent candidate was so disturbed by the numerous inquiries which the audience made as to his views in relation to current questions of local sanitation, that he cried out in despair, *"Sanitas sanitatum, et omnia sanitas!"*

III

THE AWAKENING IN AMERICA

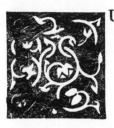URING the score of years that the great awakening of the people of England to the value of cleanliness of the individual, the home, and the municipality, as the true remedial measure against foreign as well as domestic pestilences was in progress, extending from 1846 to 1866, the people of the United States remained profoundly *Apathy in the* apathetic in relation to all *United States* questions of improvement of the public health and the prevention of epidemics.   Cholera ravaged their cities in 1849, and again in 1854, without meeting other obstruction than the occasional fumes of sulphur.   Days of fasting and prayer were religiously observed; but, for the most part, the terror-stricken people fled to the country to escape what they believed to be inevitable death if they remained in their town homes.

The object lesson which the people of England had learned from the experience of one town, and had so successfully applied in several

visitations of epidemics, was known to a few
students of sanitary science and administration
in different parts of this country, and efforts
had been made by them from time to time to
awaken public interest in sanitation of the home
and the municipality; but very little progress
was made. A few cities had health organizations, which for the most part were devoted to
political schemes and purposes, with no pretense to knowledge of the objects or methods
of sanitation.

AS the simple suggestion of the Prime Minister, that cleanliness of the home and its surroundings was the best measure of protection against cholera, contained the germ of
practical sanitary reform in England, so an incident in the writer's experience
An Incident   became the potential force that
That Counted gave to New York a most complete system of health laws and
ordinances, and an efficient administrative department of health. In a larger sense it may
with justice be claimed that this incident contained the germ of health reform that has given
to this entire country the most perfect system
of municipal, state, and national health administration in the civilized world.

The incident referred to occurred in the fifties
of the last century. New York was in the grip
of the deadly typhus. This was sometimes called

the "Spotted Fever," from the dark spots which appeared on the body of its victims, and also "Emigrant Fever," because it was brought to this country by the immigrants, especially by those who came from Ireland. Indeed, the Irish immigrants suffered so generally and severely that the disease was sometimes called the "Irish Fever." Immigration from Ireland was at that time at its flood, and the typhus was so prevalent among these poverty-stricken people that the hospitals were overcrowded by them, and large numbers were treated in tents, both on Blackwell's Island and at the quarantine grounds on Staten Island.

Having completed a two years' term of service on the interne medical staff of Bellevue Hospital, where large numbers of typhus cases were treated, I was placed in charge of the tents on Blackwell's Island by the Commissioners of Charities. Soon after entering upon the service, I noticed that patients were continually admitted from a single building in East Twenty-second Street.

IMPRESSED with the importance of closing this fever-nest, I visited the tenement, and was not surprised at the large number of cases of fever which it furnished our hospital. It is difficult to describe the scene that the interior of the house presented to the visitor. The building was in an extreme state of dilapidation

generally; the doors and windows were broken;
the cellar was partly filled with filthy
A Fever sewage; the floors were littered with
Nest decomposing straw, which the occupants used for bedding; every
available place, from cellar to garret, was
crowded with immigrants — men, women, and
children. The whole establishment was reeking with filth, and the atmosphere was heavy
with the sickening odor of the deadly typhus,
which reigned supreme in every room.

The necessity of immediately closing this
house to further occupation by immigrants, until
it was thoroughly cleansed and made decently
habitable, was imperative, and I made inquiries
for the responsible owner. I found that the
house was never visited by anyone who claimed
to be either agent or owner; but that it was the
resort of vagrants, especially of the most recent
and destitute immigrants; that they came and
went without let or hindrance, generally remaining until attacked by the prevailing epidemic of
fever, when they were removed to the fever
hospital.

AFTER considerable inquiry in the neighbor
hood I found a person who was the real
agent of the landlord; but no other information could be obtained than that the owner took
no interest in the property, and that the agent
was under instructions not to reveal the owner's

name. A suggestion to this agent, to have the house vacated and put in good **The Unknown** condition for tenants, was **Owner** refused with a contemptuous remark as to the absurdity of furnishing such vagrants and immigrants better quarters in which to live.

As there was no Health Department to which an appeal could be made, the Metropolitan Police Department was visited and the matter laid before its president, Mr. Acton. He directed the secretary, Mr. Hawley, a lawyer, to examine the health laws and ordinances to determine what measures were in the power of the police to enforce. A search was made, and the result was that neither law nor ordinance under which the police could take action was found. Mr. Acton advised that the tax lists be examined, to find who paid taxes on the property, and thus discover the responsible party to its ownership, and then that appeal be made directly to him to authorize the necessary improvements. An examination of the tax list revealed that the owner was a wealthy man, living in an aristocratic neighborhood, a member of one of the most popular churches of the city.

The condition of his tenement house was brought to his attention, and its menace to the public health as a fruitful fever nest was explained. He was very angry at what he declared was an interference with the management of his property, and asserted, in the most emphatic manner, that as the house yielded him no rent, he would not expend a dollar for the benefit of the miserable creatures who had so wrecked the building.

With the failure of this appeal to the owner, I had exhausted, apparently, every legal and moral means of abating a nuisance dangerous to life and detrimental to health.

I N this extremity I visited the office of the *Evening Post* and explained the matter to Mr. William Cullen Bryant, then editor of that newspaper. He was at once interested in the failure of the power of the City Government to remedy such a flagrant evil. In the absence of laws and ordinances, Mr. Bryant proposed to make the case public in all of its details, and for that purpose suggested that the police should cause the arrest of the delinquent owner, and he would send a reporter to make notes of the case. A charge was made against the landlord, and he was required to appear at the Jefferson Market Court. On entering the court he was confronted by the reporter, pad and pencil in hand, who pressed him with questions as to his tenement house.

Fear of Publicity

Greatly alarmed at his situation, the owner inquired as to the purpose of the reporter, and was informed that Mr. Bryant intended to publish the proceedings of the court in the *Evening Post,* and to expose his maintenance of a fever nest of the worst description. He begged that no further proceedings be taken, and promised the court that he would immediately make all necessary improvements. He promptly vacated the house, and made such a thorough reconstruction of the entire establishment that it became one of the most attractive tenements in that East Side district. For many years that house continued to be entirely free from the ordinary contagious diseases of the tenement houses of the city. It is an interesting fact that the landlord subsequently thanked the writer for having compelled him to improve his tenement house; for he had secured first-class tenants who paid him high rents.

THIS incident came to the attention of several prominent citizens, physicians, lawyers, and clergymen, who became profoundly impressed with the revelation that there were no laws under which such a glaring violation of the simplest principles of health, and even of common decency, could be at once corrected.

Agitation for Reform

For many years there had been a growing sentiment in favor of a reform of our health regulations, stimulated by the writings of Dr. John H. Griscom, Dr. Joseph M. Smith, Dr. Elisha Harris, and others, and the Academy of

Medicine had occasionally passed resolutions favoring adequate health laws; but no results had
been secured.

It was now resolved to organize a society
devoted expressly to sanitary reform, and the
"Sanitary Association" came into existence. For
several years this body annually introduced a
health bill into the Legislature, but the measure
was regularly defeated through the active opposition of the City Inspector, whose office would
be abolished if the bill became a law.

IN the early sixties the famous "Citizens Association" was organized, with Peter Cooper
as President, and a membership of one hundred of the most prominent citizens. This was
in the days of the Tweed régime, and at a period
when the City Government was
most completely in his power.
The objects of the Association
were reform in all branches of
the Municipal Government, the promotion of
wise legislation, and the defeat of all attempts
to subordinate the city to the schemes for control by Tweed and the coterie of politicians who
were under his directions.

The friends of sanitary reform decided to attempt to secure proper legislation through the
Citizens Association. The application, by a dele-
gation, for the aid of this Association was well
received and a plan of procedure adopted. The

*The Citizens
Association*

secretary of the Citizens Association, Mr. Nathaniel Sands, had been a member of the Sanitary Association, and as an enthusiastic sanitarian had been disappointed at its repeated failure to secure legislation. At his suggestion, it was decided to create two committees, one on health and another on law, and through these agencies to have the Citizens Association accomplish its work. The first committee eventually came under my direction, while the second was directed by Dorman B. Eaton, Esq.

In the Committee on Public Health were many of the more prominent medical men of that period, as Dr. Valentine Mott, Dr. Joseph M. Smith, Dr. James R. Wood, Prof. John W. Draper, Dr. Willard Parker, Dr. Isaac E. Taylor. The Committee on Law was equally distinguished for its membership, having on its list the names of William M. Evarts, Charles Tracy, D. B. Silliman.

IT was determined, as a preliminary step, to prepare a "Health Bill" and introduce it into the Legislature, which was that of 1864, and thus learn the obstacles to be met; for efforts had repeatedly been made to pass health bills without success. The bill was drawn *A Health* along the lines of previous bills, and *Bill* was altogether inadequate in its provisions to effect the required reforms. The effort, however, developed the fact

that the real opposition to health legislation was
the City Inspector's Department. As that department exercised all of the health powers, any
proper health bill would abolish it altogether.
The City Inspector, at that time, was a grossly
ignorant politician, but as he had upwards of
one million of dollars at his disposal, he had a
prevailing influence in the Legislature when
any bill affected his interests. At the hearing
on the Association's bill, the City Inspector's
agents denied every allegation as to the unsanitary condition of the city, and as the Association
had no definite information as to the facts asserted, the bill failed, as had all the bills of the
Sanitary Association during the previous ten
years.

I N conference it was now decided to make a
thorough sanitary inspection of the city by
a corps of competent physicians, draft a new
and much more comprehensive measure, and
thus be prepared to confront the City Inspector
with reliable facts in
Sanitary Inspection   regard to the actual
of New York   condition of the city.
The Citizens' Associa-
tion consented to bear the expense of the undertaking.

Under the auspices of the Association, and in
the absence of the secretary of the Committee
on Health, Dr. Elisha Harris, who was at that

time in the service of the United States Sanitary Association, I organized and supervised the inspection. The corps of inspectors consisted of young physicians, each assigned to one of the districts into which the city was divided. The work was completed during the summer months of 1864, and the original reports of the inspectors were bound in seventeen large folio volumes. These reports were afterwards edited by the secretary, Dr. Elisha Harris, and published by the Association in a volume of over 500 pages. The total cost to the Association of this inspection and publication was $22,000; but it richly repaid the Association, for it accomplished the object for which it was undertaken.

This volunteer sanitary inspection of a great city was regarded by European health authorities as the most remarkable and creditable in the history of municipal reform. Too much credit can not be given to the President of the Association, Peter Cooper, and to the Secretary, Nathaniel Sands, for the constant support which they gave the Committee on Health in the prosecution of this great undertaking.

Meantime the Committee on Law perfected a bill to be introduced at the coming session of the Legislature, 1865. It was the joint product of the Medical and Law Committees, and was made the subject of extensive study and research, in order to embody in it every provision essential to its practical operations.

At the request of the Committees I made the
first draft for the purpose of embodying the
sanitary features as the basis of the bill. Former
health bills ·were restricted in their operations
to the city of New York, and the officers were
appointed by the Mayor. As the government
of the city was dominated in all of its departments by Tweed, it was decided to place the
proposed new health organization under the
control of the State, by making a Metropolitan
Health District, the area of which should be
co-extensive with that of the Metropolitan Police District. This feature of the bill was also
important because the protection of the city
from contagious diseases in outlying districts
required that the jurisdiction of the Board
should extend to contiguous populations.

The original draft having been approved by
the Committee on Health, Mr. Eaton was re-
quested to perfect the bill by adding the legal
provisions. As he had recently made a study of
the English health laws, he incorporated many
items especially relating to the powers of the
Board which were quite novel in this country.

ONE feature of the bill deserves mention; for
it is an anomaly in legislation and apparently violates the most sacred principle of
justice; viz., the power of the courts to review
the proceedings of a health board. The Committees concluded that a board which was au-

thorized to abate nuisances "dangerous to life
and detrimental to health" should
An Anomaly not be subjected to the possible
in Law liability of being interrupted in
its efforts to abate them by
an injunction that would delay its action. Accordingly the law as so drawn that the Metropolitan Board was empowered to create ordinances, to execute them in its own time and
manner, and to sit in judgment on its own acts,
without the possibility of being interrupted by
review proceedings or injunctions by any court.
Its power was made autocratic. The language
of that portion of the bill conveying these powers was purposely made very technical, in order
that only a legal mind could interpret its full
meaning, it being believed that the ordinary
legislator would not favor the measure if he
understood its entire import. It is an interesting fact that the first case brought into court
under the law was an effort to prove the uncon-
stitutionality of this feature; but it was carried
to the Court of Appeals, and its constitutional-
ity was sustained by a majority of one.

ON the assembling of the Legislature of 1865
the Metropolitan Health Bill was formally
introduced into both houses, and preparations made to secure its passage. Mr. Eaton was
selected by the Citizens' Association to advocate
the legal provisions of the bill at the hearings

before the committees of the Legislature, and I
was delegated to explain
Introduction of an the sanitary requirements
Epoch-Making Bill of the measure. The first
hearing occurred on the
thirteenth of February, before a joint committee of both houses, Hon. Andrew D. White,
senator, presiding. A large audience was present, including the City Inspector and the usual
retinue of office holders in his department. The
Citizens Association was represented by Rev.
Henry W. Bellows, Dr. James R. Wood, Dr.
Willard Parker, Prof. John W. Draper, and several other prominent citizens, in addition to Mr.
Eaton and myself.

Mr. Eaton first addressed the committee, and
made an admirable presentation of the legal
features of the bill. He eloquently appealed
for its enactment into law, in order to create
in New York a competent health authority, with
power to relieve the city of its gross sanitary
evils and adopt and enforce measures for the
promotion of the public health.

I followed him, my task being to show, from
the existing condition of the city, the imperative
need of such legislation. My remarks on the
occasion were published in *The New York
Times* of March 16, 1865.

IV

NEW YORK, THE UNCLEAN

The illustrations in this chapter, with the front-ispiece of the book, have all been reproduced from the elaborate report published by the Council of Hygiene of the Citizens' Association. My address before the Legislative Committee is here given as it then appeared in *The New York Times* of March 13, 1865, with the correction of some typographical errors. It consisted of a detailed presentation of the facts recorded and sworn to by the medical inspectors employed by the Citizens' Association, together with photographic illustrations which were made by them.

R. CHAIRMAN: I have been requested to lay before you some of the results of a sanitary inspection of New York City, undertaken and prosecuted to a successful completion by a voluntary organization of citizens. There has long been a settled conviction in the minds of the medical men of New York, that

Alarm of Medical Men
that city is laboring under sanitary evils of which it might be relieved. This opinion is not mere conjecture, but it is based upon the daily observations which they are accustomed to make in the pursuit of professional duties.

Familiar, by daily study, with the causes of diseases, and the laws which govern their spread, they have seen yearly accumulating about and within the homes of the laboring classes all the recognized causes of the most preventible diseases, without a solitary measure being taken by those in authority to apply an effectual remedy. They have seen the poor

crowded into closer and closer quarters, until
the system has actually become one of tenant-
house packing. They have witnessed the prevalence of terrible and fatal epidemics, having
their origin in or intensified by these conditions,
and many of their professional brethren have
perished in the courageous performance of
their duties to the poor and suffering.

Cognizant of these growing evils, and believing that they are susceptible of removal, they
have repeatedly and publicly protested against
the longer tolerance of such manifest causes of
disease and death in our city. Large bodies of
influential citizens have been equally impressed
with the importance of radical reform in the
health organizations of New York, and have
strenuously labored, but in vain, to obtain
proper legislative enactments.

TO give practical effect to their efforts, it was
determined in May last to undertake a systematic investigation of the sanitary condition of the city. For this purpose a central organization was formed, and when I mention the
names of its leading members, I
give you the best assurance that
the work was undertaken in the
interests of science and human-
ity. The president was Dr. Joseph M. Smith,
one of the ablest writers on sanitary science in
this country, and among its members were

*A Systematic
Investigation*

Drs. Valentine Mott, James Anderson, Willard
Parker, Alonzo Clark, Gurdon Buck, James R.
Wood, Charles Henschel, Alfred C. Post, Isaac
E. Taylor, John W. Draper, R. Ogden Doremus,
Henry Goulden, Henry D. Bulkley, and Elisha
Harris.

In prosecuting this inquiry the Association
was guided by the experience of similar organizations in Great Britain, where sanitary science
is now cultivated with the greatest zeal, and is
yielding the richest fruits. As a preliminary
step to the introduction of sanitary reforms,
many of the populous towns of England made
a more or less complete inspection of the homes
of the people to determine their condition, and
to enable them to arrive at correct conclusions
as to the required remedial measures. The
English Government undertook a similar investigation through its "Commissioners for In-
quiring into the State of Large Towns and
Populous Districts," and the voluminous and
exhaustive reports of that Commission laid the
foundation of the admirable sanitary system of
that country.

The first object of sanitary organization was
apparently, therefore, to obtain detailed information as to the existing causes of disease
and the mortality of the population, and as to
the special incidence of that mortality upon each sex, and each age, on separate places,
on various occupations; in fact, to present

a detailed account of what may be called, in
commercial phrase, our transactions in human
life.

E VIDENTLY the best method of arriving at
  such knowledge was by a systematic in-
    spection. And that inspection must be a
house-to-house visitation, in which the course
of inquiry not only developed all the facts relating to the sanitary, but
A House-to-House   equally to the social con-
Inspection   dition of the people. It
must necessarily be re-
quired of the inspector that he visit every house,
and every family in the house, and learn by
personal examination, inquiry, and observation,
every circumstance, external and internal to the
domicile, bearing upon the health of the individual.

To perform such service satisfactorily, skilled
labor must be employed. No student of general
science, much less a common artisan, was qualified to undertake this investigation into the
causes of disease; however patent these causes
might be, he had no power to appreciate their
real significance. Minds trained by education,
and long experience in observing and treating
the diseases of the laboring classes, could alone
thoroughly and properly accomplish the work
proposed.

HAPPILY, experts were at hand and prepared to enter upon the task, viz.: the dispensary physicians. The daily duties of these practitioners have been for years to practice among the poor, and study minutely their diseases; and thus they have gained an

The Medical Experts extensive and accurate knowledge of the sanitary and social condition of the mass of the people. Many of these practitioners have been engaged in dispensary service, and in a single district, for ten to twenty years. They have thus become so familiar with the poor of their district, though often numbering 40,000 to 50,000, that they know the peculiarities of each house, the class of disease prevalent each month of the year, and to a large extent the habits, character, etc., of the families which occupy them.

From this class of medical men the Council selected, as far as possible, its corps of Inspectors. As a body, they represent the best medical talent of the junior portion of the profession of New York. Many occupy high social positions, and all were men of refinement, education, and devotion to duty. They entered upon the work with the utmost enthusiasm; engaging in it as a purely scientific study.

Everywhere the people welcomed the Inspectors, invited them to examine their homes, and gave them the most ample details.

T HE plan of inspection adopted by the Council was as follows: The city was divided into thirty-one districts and an Inspector selected for each, care being taken to assign to each inspector a district with which he was most familiar. The Inspector was directed

Plan of Inspection to commence his inspection by first traversing the whole district, to learn its general and topographical peculiarities. He was then to take up the squares in detail, examining them consecutively as they lie in belts.

Commencing at a given corner of his district, he was first to go around the square and note: 1. Nature of the ground. 2. Drainage and sewerage. 3. Number of houses in the square. 4. Vacant lots and their sanitary condition. 5. Courts and alleys. 6. Rear buildings. 7. Number of tenement houses. 11. Drinking shops, brothels, gambling saloons, etc. 12. Stores and markets. 13. Factories, schools, crowded buildings. 14. Slaughter-houses (describe particularly). 15. Bone and offal nuisances. 16. Stables, etc. 17. Churches and school edifices.

Returning to the point of starting, he was to commence a detailed inspection of each building, noting: *a.* Condition and material of buildings. *b.* Number of stories and their height. *c.* Number of families intended to be accommodated, and space allotted to each. *d.* Water supply and house drainage. *e.* Location and character of water-closets. *f*. Disposal of garbage and house slops. *g*. Ventilation, external and internal. *h*. Cellars and basements, and their population. *i*. Conditions of halls and passages. *j*. Frontage on street, court, alley — N., E., S. or W. 18. Prevailing character of the population. 19. Prevailing sickness and mortality. 20. Sources of preventible disease and mortality. 21. Condition of streets and pavements. 22. Miscellaneous information.

H E entered each room, examined its means of ventilation and its contents, noted the number of occupants by day and by night, and carefully estimated the cubical area to each person. Whenever any contagious or infectious disease was discovered, as *Each Room* fever, smallpox, measles, scar-*Examined* latina, the Inspector made a special report upon the dwelling. This report embodied specific answers to a series of questions, furnished in a blank form, requiring him 1. To trace and record the medical history of the sick person. 2. To ascertain and record facts relating to the family and other persons exposed to the patients and to the causes of the malady. 3. To report the sanitary condition of the domicil. 4. To report the statistics and sanitary condition of the population of that domicil. 5. To report upon the sanitary condition of the locality or neighborhood and

its population. 6. To preserve and make returns of these records. 7. To prepare on the
spot the necessary outlines or data for the
sketching of a map or descriptive chart of the
domicil, block, or locality.

Each Inspector was supplied with a note-
book and a permanent record-book; in the first
he constantly made notes as his examination
proceeded, and in the latter these notes were
expanded and put on permanent record. These
permanent record-books are the property of
the Association and embrace for the most part
minute details concerning every building and
tenement occupied by the laboring classes, as
also, grog-shops, stables, vacant lots, slaughter-
houses, etc.

Each Inspector was furnished with materials
for drawing, and was directed to make accurate
drawings of the squares in his district, locating
each building, vacant lot, etc., and distinguishing the character and condition of each by an
appropriate color. Many of these drafts of
districts are beautiful specimens of art, and as
sanitary charts enable the observer to locate infectious and contagious diseases, and with the
aid of the permanent records, to determine the
internal and external domiciliary conditions
under which they occur.

I have been thus minute in specifying the details of the plan of inspection, the qualifications
of the Inspectors, and the means employed, in

order that the character of the work and the
value of the results obtained may be properly
appreciated.

E ARLY in the month of May the work of thoroughly inspecting the insalubrious quarters,
where fever and other pestilential diseases
prevail, had been commenced, and the fact was
soon ascertained that smallpox and typhus fever were existing and spreading
Period of the in almost every crowded lo-
Inspection cality of the city. It was not
until about the middle of July
that the entire corps of Inspectors was engaged.
The work was then prosecuted with vigor and
without interruption to the middle of November, when it was completed. The Inspectors
met regularly every Saturday evening to report
to a committee on the part of the Council the
progress of their work, and to receive advice
and instruction in regard to all questions of a
doubtful character.

On the completion of the inspection each Inspector was required to prepare a final report
embodying the general results of his labors.
These reports have all been properly collated,
under the direction of the Association, and are
now passing through the press. They will soon
appear in an octavo volume of about 400 pages,
largely illustrated, with maps and diagrams. It
will be the first interior view of the sanitary and

social condition of the population of New York, and will abundantly demonstrate the fact that, though a great and prosperous commercial centre, she does not afford happy homes to hundreds of thousands.

B EFORE proceeding to an analysis of this work, it will be necessary to notice the topographical peculiarities of our city, and the distribution of its population. New York is an island having an area of about thirty-four square miles, inclusive of its *Distribution of* parks. Unlike Philadelphia, *Population* London, and most other large cities, which have a background of hundreds of square miles upon which to extend according to the exigencies of the population or of business, New York is limited in its power of expansion, and must accomodate itself to its given area. While it is true that a large business population will gather upon the adjacent shores, it is equally true that these non-residents will be of the better class. The laboring population will, for the most part, remain upon the island, and must be accommodated in the city proper, as they are compelled to live near their work.

New York has, thus far, grown without any control or supervision, until its population is estimated at 1,000,000 of persons. Of this number, at least one-half are of the laboring and de-

pendant classes, compelled to live under such
conditions as they find in their homes, without
any power, either to change or improve them.
Following the natural law which governs the
movements of such a population, the wealthier
or independent class spreads itself with its business arrangements over the larger proportion
of the area, and the poorer or dependent class
is crowded into the smallest possible space.

ALREADY New York has covered about 8 of
its 34 square miles with the dwellings of a
population not far from 1,000,000, and all
its commercial and manufacturing establishments.   And the result is, as might have been
anticipated,   the   dependent
class, numbering fully one-
half of the people, is crowded
into tenant-houses which oc-
cupy an area of not more than two square
miles.   Such crowding amounts literally to
packing.

Tenant-House Packing

For example, it is estimated that there are
three contiguous blocks of tenant-houses which
contain a larger population than Fifth Avenue;
or, again, if Fifth Avenue had front and rear
tenant-houses as densely packed as tenant-
houses generally are, there would be a population of 100,000 on that single avenue.   A single
tenant-court in the Fourth Ward is arranged
for the packing of 1,000 persons.

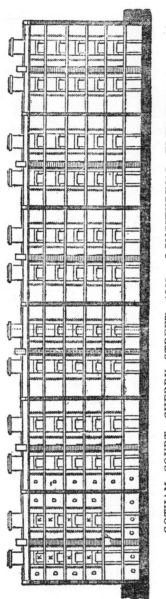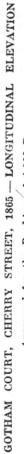

GOTHAM COURT, CHERRY STREET, 1865 — LONGITUDINAL ELEVATION

Arranged for the Packing of 1,000 Persons

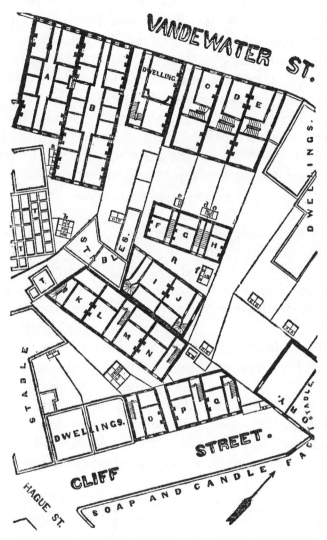

SECTION OF CITY 240 BY 150 FEET, OCCUPIED
BY 111 FAMILIES, AND BY STABLES, SOAP
FACTORY, AND TANYARD

A resident of the same Ward reports that: "On a piece of ground 240 feet by 150, there are 20 tenant-houses, occupied by 111 families, 5 stables, a large soap and candle factory, and a tan-yard, the receptacle of green hides. The filth and stench of this locality are beyond any power of description." In general, it may be stated that the average number of families to a house among the poor is 7, or about 35 persons.

IT is necessary also to make a single explanation, to render more apparent the bearing of the facts developed. For the purposes of sanitary inquiry, the causes of disease are divided into those which are inevitable, and those which are avoidable or re-movable, and hence it follows that diseases and deaths are divided into those which are inevitable and those which are preventable. For example: Of unavoidable causes of disease, we have vicissitudes of weather, accidents, old age, physical degenerations, etc.

Avoidable and Inevitable Disease

Of avoidable or removable causes of disease we have those conditions around or within our dwellings or places of business or resort, errors in our mode of living, etc., which vitiate health, or rather tend to diseases, and yet which can be removed or changed by human agency. For example, a country residence may be most favorably located for health, and yet decaying vegetable matter in the cellar, or a cesspool so situated as to allow the gaseous emanations to be diffused through the house, will expose all the inmates to fevers, diarrhœa and dysentery. These would be preventable diseases, and all the deaths therefrom would be preventable, and hence unnecessary deaths. In like manner in cities, all diseases and deaths due to causes which human agencies can remove are preventable. And it is a melancholy fact that fifty per cent of the mortality of cities is estimated to be due to such causes, and is hence unnecessary.

In reviewing the result of this inspection, I shall call your attention only to the more patent causes of disease found existing, and to the preventable diseases discovered, and their relation to these causes. In this evidence you will find ample proof that radical reforms are required in the health organizations of New York.

I WILL first notice the causes of disease which exist external to our dwellings, and which are the most readily susceptible of remedy. The first that attracts attention in New York is the condition of the streets. No one can *Filthy* doubt that if the streets in a thickly *Streets* populated part of a town are made the common receptacle of the refuse of families, that in its rapid decomposition a vast amount of poisonous gases must escape, which will impregnate the entire district, penetrate the dwellings, and render the atmosphere in the neighborhood in a high degree injurious to the public health. In confirmation of this statement, I will quote the City Inspector, who, in a former communication to the Common Council, says:

"As an evidence of the effect of this state of things upon the health of the community, I would state that the mortality of the city, from the first of March, has been largely on the increase, until it has now reached a point of fearful magnitude. For the week ending April 27th, there were reported to this department one hundred and forty more deaths than occurred during the same week of the previous year. Were this increase of mortality the result of an existing pestilence or epidemic among us, the public would become justly alarmed as to the future; but although no actual pestilence, as such, exists, it is by no means certain that we are not preparing the way for some fatal scourge by the no longer to be endured filthy condition of our city."

The universal testimony of the sanitary inspectors is that in all portions of the city occupied by the poorer classes, the streets are in the same filthy condition as that described by the City Inspector, and, that street filth is one of the most fruitful causes of disease.

SAYS the Inspector of the Eighth Ward: "Laurens, Wooster, Clark, and Sullivan are in a most filthy condition, giving off insalubrious emanations on which depend the many cases of fever, cholera infantum, dysentery, and pulmonary diseases. I have *Street Filth* observed that near where other *and Disease* streets cross the above-named streets there is a greater proportionate amount of sickness; and this fact I have shown by special reports of typhus and typhoid fever in Grand and Broome, and dysentery in Spring."

The Inspector of the Sixth Ward says: "Domestic garbage and filth of every kind is thrown into the streets, covering their surface, filling the gutters, obstructing the sewer culverts, and sending forth perennial emanations which must generate pestiferous disease. In winter the filth and garbage, etc., accumulate in the streets, to the depth sometimes of two or three feet. The garbage boxes are a perpetual source of nuisance in the streets, filth and offal being thrown all around them, pools of filthy water in many instances remaining in the gutters, and having their source in the garbage boxes."

The Inspector of the Seventh Ward says: "The whole most easterly portion of the district, the streets and gutters are very filthy with mud, ashes, garbage, etc."

The Inspector of the Thirteenth Ward says:

"The streets are generally in a filthy and unwholesome condition; especially in front of the tenant-houses, from which the garbage and slops are, to a great extent, thrown into the streets, where they putrefy, rendering the air offensive to the smell and deleterious to health. The refuse of the bedrooms of those sick with typhoid and scarlet fevers and smallpox is frequently thrown into the streets, there to contaminate the air, and, no doubt, aid in the spread of those pestilential diseases."

Says the Inspector of the Ninth Ward: "The effect of dirty streets upon the public health is too well known, and too often insisted upon, to need any exposition in this report. The largest number of cases of cholera infantum, cholera morbus, and kindred disease, is always found in localities where the streets are dirtiest."

The Inspector of the Seventeenth Ward writes: "The two following localities present the appearance of dung-hills rather than the thoroughfares in a civilized city, viz.: Sixth Street, between Bowery and Second Avenue, and Eleventh Street, between First and Second Avenues."

THE Inspector of the Eleventh Ward says: "As a rule, the streets are extremely dirty and offensive, and the gutters obstructed with filth. The filth of the streets is composed of house-slops, refuse vegetables, decayed fruit, store and shop sweepings, ashes, dead animals, and even human excrements. These *Animals Dead* putrifying organic substances are ground together by the constantly passing vehicles. When dried by the summer's heat, they are driven by the wind in every direction in the form of dust. When remaining moist or liquid in the form of "slush," they emit deleterious and very offensive exhalations.. The reeking stench of the gutters, the street filth, and domestic garbage of this quarter of the city, constantly imperil the health of its inhabitants. It is a well-recognized cause of diarrhoeal diseases and fevers."

The Inspector of the Eighteenth Ward reports: "The streets in the eastern part of the district, east of First Avenue especially, have, for the past six months, been in a most inexcusably filthy condition. The pavement here is uneven, there are deep gutters at either side of the streets, filled with foul slops, in which float or are sunk every form of decaying animal and vegetable matter. Occasionally, at remote and irregular intervals, carts come round, these stagnant pools are dredged, so to speak, and their black and decayed solid contents raked out. If there be anything on earth that is 'rank and smells to heaven,' these gutters do on such occasions, especially in the summer months. The streets in this part of the city are the principal depositories of garbage. In some instances

heaped up at the sides of the streets, in others
thrown about promiscuously, the event in either
case is the same, if it be allowed to remain day
after day, as it usually is. After having passed
through every stage of decay, after having cor-
rupted the surrounding air with its pestilential
smell, it gradually becomes dessicated and converted into dust by the summer sun and the
constantly passing vehicles. And now every
horse that passes stirs it up, every vehicle leaves
a cloud of it behind; it is lifted into the air with
every wind and carried in every direction.

"Those who are directly responsible for this
state of things suffer no more than the cleanly
and thrifty who are so unfortunate as to live
anywhere the wind, blowing from this quarter,
reaches them. And what a *pulvis compositum*
is it to breathe into the lungs! As we pass by,
our mouths become full of it, we draw it in with
our breath. It is swallowed into the stomach,
it penetrates our dress and clings until it
has covered our perspiring skin. Surely no
dumping-ground, no sewer, no vault, contains
more filth or in greater variety than did the air
in certain parts of our city during the long season of drought the past summer. And wherever
the wind blows, the foul corruption is carried;
by a process as sure and universal as the diffusion of gases, is it conveyed throughout the city.
Such, often, is the air drawn into the lungs with
every respiration,, of the poor sufferer stifled

with consumption or burning with fever. No barrier can shut it out, no social distinction can save us from it; no domestic cleanliness, no private sanitary measures can substitute a pure atmosphere for a foul one."

But I need not multiply these quotations. It will suffice to state that during the week ending August 5th, a special inspection of all the streets was made and they were found to be reeking, and, indeed, almost impassable, with filth. And to-day they are in, if possible, a still worse condition than ever before.

CLOSELY allied to the streets are courts and alleys. These cul-de-sacs leading to, and adjoining the close and unventilated homes of the poor, are almost universally in a more filthy condition than the adjacent street. They are the receptacles of much of *Filthy Courts* the waste of the house, and are *and Alleys* rarely cleaned. The air of these places during the summer is often the most stifling and irrespirable, and yet as it descends it enters the closely packed tenant-house and furnishes to the inmates the elements of disease and death. Says the Inspector of the Fourth Ward:

"Slops from rear buildings of such premises are usually emptied into a shallow gutter cut in the flagging and extending from the yard, or space between front and rear buildings, to the

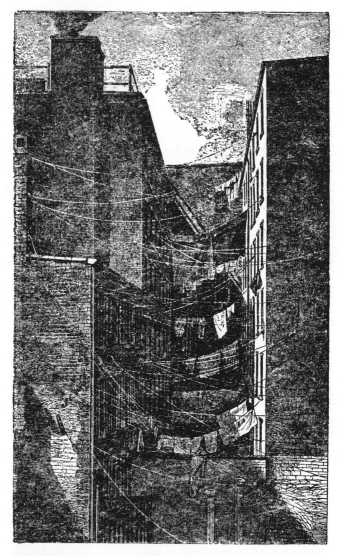

A TENANT-HOUSE CUL-DE-SAC, PARK STREET, NEAR
CITY HALL, WITH 307 INMATES; PHOTOGRAPHED
FROM A HOUSE-TOP IN PEARL STREET, 1865

street.   This is often clogged up by semi-fluid
filth, so that the alley and those parts of the
yard through which it runs are not infrequently
overflown and submerged to the depth of several inches.   There are more than four hundred
families in this district whose homes can only
be reached by wading through a disgusting deposit of filthy refuse.   In some instances, a stag-

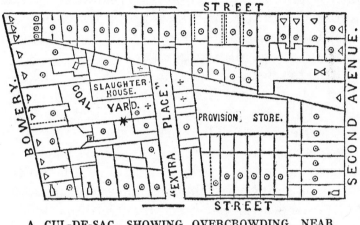

A CUL-DE-SAC, SHOWING OVERCROWDING, NEAR
SLAUGHTER-HOUSE AND STABLES
New York, 1865

ing of plank, elevated a few inches above the
surface, is constructed through the alleys."

I N the court is found generally that most
pestiferous of all the sources of civic unclean-
liness and unhealthiness — the privy and
cesspool.   These receptacles are rarely drained
into the sewers, and consequently require for

their cleanliness the frequent and faithful attention of the scavenger.   The re-
Cesspool   ports of the sanitary inspectors
Abominations   prove that this work is most
irregularly   and   imperfectly
done.   Hundreds of places were found where
these nuisances existed within, under or beside
large tenant-houses, creating a vast amount of
disease and death.   Numerous instances of this
kind are detailed in these reports, which are almost too revolting to be believed.   I will quote
but one or two illustrations:

"The privies (two in one) of Nos. — and —
West Twenty-fourth Street need instant cleaning.   They are overflowing the yard, and are
very offensive.   The privy No. — Seventh
Avenue, as in the preceding two adjoining
houses, is in the yard, and adjoins the house,
and is on a line with the southerly wall of house
No. — (the adjacent house), which has a back
area; the wall of said area being part of the
foundation of the privy.   At times the fluid portion of the privy oozes through its own and the
area wall.

"The privy of the rear tenant-house No. —
West Twenty-second Street is used by 42 persons; it has five subdivisions, one for every two
families.   The compartments are so small that
a person can scarcely turn round in them, and
so dark that they have to be entered with an
artificial light.   The cellar itself, as has been

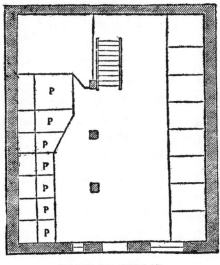

PLAN OF CELLAR

stated, is damp, dark, and without ventilation. Under such circumstances the emanations of the excrementious matter of 42 persons can find no escape; thus this privy-cellar is worse than a Stygian pit."

The Inspector of the Fifth Ward says: "Very few tenements have water-closets in the house; they have privies in the yards, which, as a rule, are insufficient for the accommodation of the numbers crowded into the houses; many are not connected with the sewers; are seldom cleaned, being allowed to overflow in some cases, rendering the neighborhood offensive with insalubrious emanations."

The Inspector of the Fourteenth Ward states that: "The water-closets are nearly all in the yards — but few being in the houses — and connecting with the sewers. The greater number of these sewers are in a filthy condition, being but seldom emptied. Many of those which communicate with the privies are choked up by all sorts of offal being thrown into them, thereby producing a very bad condition."

THE Inspector of the Seventeenth Ward reports: "The privies of East Eleventh Street, rear, are beneath the floored alley-way leading to the building. Large holes in this floor allow ocular inspection from above, and admit rain and dirt. These nuisances *Unbelievable* are almost always overflowing, *Vileness* and the passage leading to them is full of fæcal matter. It would seem impossible for human beings to create or endure such vileness. The cellar is used by children and others as a privy; the foul air there seems never to change."

The Inspector of the Sixteenth Ward says: "The privies form one end of the chief features of insalubrity. Nearly all of them are too small in size and too few in number, and without ventilation or seat-covers. About twelve were found locked securely, and on procuring the key and inspecting the privy, such masses of human excrements were found on the seats and floors as would justify the locking of the door to protect unwary persons from injury. Occupants of rear buildings are the principal sufferers from this insalubrity. The proximity of privies is in some cases eight feet from the windows of rear houses; the odor in these is, especially at night, intolerable. Instances of the kind are to

be found at Nos. —, — and — West Seventeenth
Street, and others. They are also too few in
number; for example, No. — West Nineteenth
Street, where in the front and rear buildings
more than one hundred persons live who have
one common privy, with a single partition dividing it, and but four seats in all. Twenty-five
persons are expected to use one seat-opening."

The Inspector of the Twentieth Ward says:
"During my inspection I reported a number
which were filled, and at the same time in such
need of repair as to hazard the lives of those
who entered them. The proximity of these
places to the houses in many cases is a fact to
which I would call your attention. One instance
of this kind I may state: At a house in Fortieth
Street, between Broadway and Seventh Avenue,
the privy is situated about 10 feet from the door,
and there is another on a line 10 feet from the
first, and still another within 10 feet of the last
mentioned, making three privies within 30 feet,
and two of these belong to houses fronting on
Broadway. The offensive odor arising from
these places contaminates the air of the houses
in the vicinity. This house, in Fortieth Street,
is actually unfit to live in. At the time of my
inspection the noxious gases from these privies
were strongly perceptible in every part of the
house."

The Inspector of the Seventeenth Ward reports: "The privies are in most cases in the rear

court-yard. In about two-thirds of the houses
the privies are connected with the sewer. Overflowing privies are frequently found. Sometimes they are located in a dark place, which
in all cases must be considered an evil. Such
is the case in some houses in Rivington, Stanton, Ninth and Eldridge streets. All these places
are filthy, and exceedingly offensive and dangerous to the whole neighborhood; in some
places the foundation of the privies being rotten
and broken, and fæcal matter runs into the
cellar, as in No. — 'Extra Place,' where diseases
and deaths have occurred. The contents of a
privy in a court at No. — Fifth Street have, from
a similar cause, saturated the yard of premises
on the Bowery, where several children died
during the summer."

I WILL at this point simply allude to special
nuisances. New York has within the narrow
limits of its present occupied area of about
eight square miles, in addition to its one million
of people, and all its commercial and manufacturing establishments, a vast num-
Special　　ber of special nuisances, which are,
Nuisances　to a greater or less degree, detrimental to its public health.
There are nearly 200 slaughter-houses, many of
which are in the most densely populated districts. To these places droves of cattle, hogs,
and sheep are constantly driven, rendering the

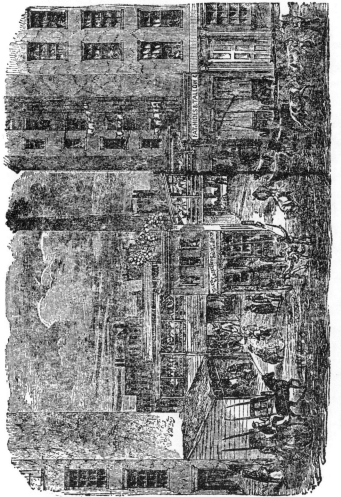

SLAUGHTER-PENS IN REAR OF TENANT-HOUSES IN THE
ELEVENTH WARD, 1865

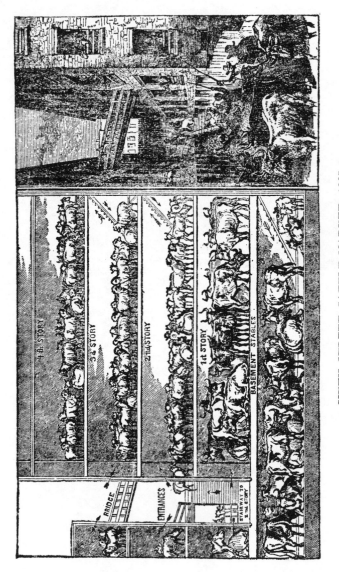

SIXTH STREET CATTLE MARKET, 1865

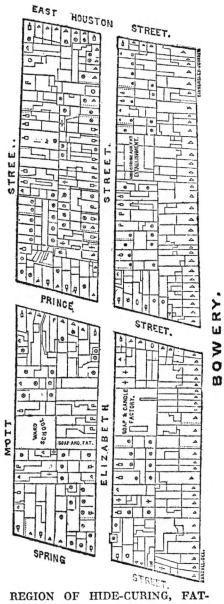

REGION OF HIDE-CURING, FAT-
GATHERING, FAT AND SOAP
BOILING, AND SLAUGHTER-PENS,
BEHIND THE BOWERY SHOPPING
HOUSES, 1865

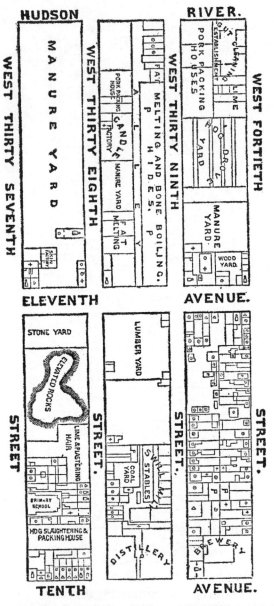

REGION OF BONE-BOILING AND SWILL-MILK
NUISANCES, 1865

streets filthy in the extreme, and from them flow
blood and refuse of the most disgusting character.

In certain populous sections are fat-boiling,
entrails-cleansing, and tripe-curing establishments, which poison the air for squares around
with their stifling emanations. To these must
be added hundreds of uncleaned stables, immense manure heaps, etc., etc. But I shall not
dwell further on these subjects, and the evidence
regarding them.

I PASS from the consideration of the external
  to the internal domiciliary conditions. The
poorer classes of New York are found living
either in cellars or in tenement houses. It is
estimated by the City Inspector that 18,000 persons live in cellars. This
Cellar Population—   is also about the es-
Dens of Death   timate of the police.
The apartments of these
people are not the light and airy basement
rooms of the better class houses, but their
homes are, in the worst sense, cellars. These
dark, damp and dreary abodes are seldom
penetrated by a ray of sunlight, or enlivened by
a breath of fresh air. I will quote several descriptions from these reports. In the Fourth
Ward many of these cellars are below tide
water. Says the Inspector of that district:
"This submarine region is not only excessively

damp, but is liable to sudden inroads from the
sea. At high tide the water often wells up
through the floors, submerging them to a considerable depth. In very many cases the vaults
of privies are situated on the same or a higher
level, and their contents frequently ooze
through the walls into the occupied apartments
beside them. Fully one-fourth of these subterranean domiciles are pervaded by a most
offensive odor from this source, and rendered
exceedingly unwholesome as human habitations. These are the places in which we most
frequently meet with typhoid fever and dysentery during the summer months. I estimate
the amount of sickness of all kinds affecting the
residents of basements and cellars, compared
with that occurring among an equal number of
the inhabitants of floors above ground, as being
about a ratio of 3 to 2."

The Inspector of the Fifteenth Ward reports:
"In a dark and damp cellar, about 18 feet square
and 7 feet high, lived a family of seven persons;
within the past year two have died of typhus,
two of smallpox, and one has been sent to the
hospital with erysipelas. The tops of the windows of this abode are below the level of the
surface, and in the court near are several privies
and a rear tenant-house. Yet this occurred but
a short distance from the very heart of the city."

The Inspector of the Ninth Ward writes: "At
Nos. —, —, — and — Hammond Street, and also

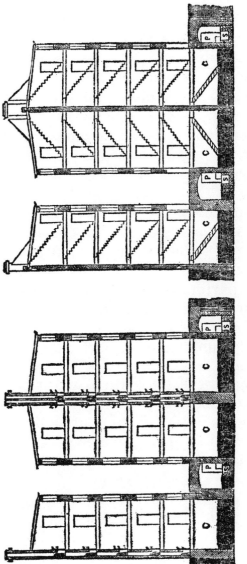

TRANSVERSE SECTIONAL ELEVATION OF THE GOTHAM COURT ROOKERY

C, CELLAR; P, PRIVY; S, SEWER

at No. — Washington Street, are inhabited cellars, the ceilings of which are below the level of the street, inaccessible to the rays of the sun, and always damp and dismal. Three of them are flooded at every heavy rain, and require to be baled out. They are let at a somewhat smaller rent than is asked for apartments on an upper floor, and are rented by those to whom poverty leaves no choice. They are rarely vacant."

The Inspector of the Seventeenth Ward states that: "In 17 squares 55 houses contain 246 persons living in cellars entirely underground. As a matter of course such cellars are unhealthy dwelling apartments. Stanton Place has some of these miserable cellar-apartments, in which diseases have been generated. These cellars are entirely subterranean, dark and damp."

THE Inspector of the Sixth Ward says: "There has been some improvement within the last few years — the cellar population having been perceptibly decreased, yet 496 persons still live in damp and unwholesome quarters under ground. In some of

496 Persons Under Ground

them water was discovered trickling down the walls, the source of which was sometimes traced to the courts and alleys, and sometimes to the soakage from the water-closets. The noxious effluvia always present in these basements are of a sickening character. Many of the cellars are occupied by two or three families; a number are also occupied as lodging-houses, accommodating from twenty to thirty lodgers. One, near the corner of Elm and Worth streets, is now fifteen or sixteen feet below the level of the street (the street having been raised ten feet). The lodging-house keeper complained to the Inspector that her business had fallen off some since the street was raised. As might be expected, the sickness rate is very high; rheumatic disease, fevers, strumous diseases, cholera infantum, etc., etc., running riot among the population. Indeed, in nearly every basement disease of some kind has been found peculiarly prevalent and fatal."

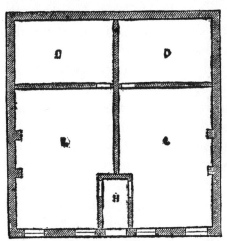

PLAN OF CELLAR IN THE SIXTEENTH WARD, 1865, OCCUPIED BY TWO FAMILIES, EACH WITH A DARK LIVING-ROOM, AND A DARK, DAMP DORMITORY

Another Inspector says: "At No. — West Sixteenth Street, two families, in which are thirteen persons, occupy the basement. It is so dark that ordinary type can be seen with difficulty. In the other case the peo-

ple were healthy before entering the basement;
since, however, they have been ill; the mother
has phthisis. Of twenty-four cellars, note of
which has been made, four only were in good
sanitary condition. The rest were more or less
filthy, some indescribably so. One contained
urine, bones, and soakage from the privy."

The Inspector of the Eighteenth Ward writes:
"There are a few cellars so dark that one cannot
see to read in them, unless by artificial light,
except for a few hours in the day, by sitting
close to the window; and there are many basement rooms into whose gloomy recesses not a
single direct ray from the sun ever shone. The
latter are, as a rule, by half their depth below
the level of the street. Dark and damp, with
very little chance for circulation of air, it would
be difficult to imagine a human being more completely beyond reach of sanitary provisions.
And when we consider that four large families
often crowd this subterranean floor, no words
are needed to show their condition deplorable.
That a generally impaired vitality is promoted
by living in this unnatural way, 'a nameless,
ever new disease,' there can be no question;
that these people will be especially prone to
whatever form of prevailing sickness may be
about in the community, no one can doubt; but
whether there is any specific cause involved,
capable of producing definite forms of disease,
is more difficult to determine."

A N Inspector thus describes a visit to one of these subterranean abodes: "We enter a room whose low ceiling is blackened with smoke, and its walls discolored with damp. In front, opening on a narrow area covered with green mould, two small windows, their tops scarcely level with the court-yard, afford at noonday a twilight illumination to the apartment. Through their broken panes they admit the damp air laden with effluvia, which constitutes the vital atmosphere inhaled by all who are immured in this dismal abode. A door at the back of this room communicates with another which is entirely dark, and has but this one opening. Both rooms together have an area of about eighteen feet square.

A Visit to the Cave-Dwellers

"The father of the family, a day laborer, is absent. The mother, a wrinkled crone at thirty, sits rocking in her arms an infant whose pasty and pallid features tell that decay and death are usurping the place of health and life. Two older children are in the street, which is their only playground, and the only place where they can go to breathe an atmosphere that is even comparatively pure. A fourth child, emaciated to a skeleton, and with that ghastly and unearthly look which marasmus impresses on its victims, has reared his feeble frame on a rickety chair against the window sill, and is striving to get a glimpse of the smiling heavens, whose

light is so seldom permitted to gladden its long-
ing eyes. Its youth has battled nobly against
the terrible morbid and devitalizing agents
which have oppressed its childish life — the
poisonous air, the darkness, and the damp; but
the battle is nearly over — it is easy to decide
where the victory will be."

But I need not multiply the evidences that
18,000 people, men, women, and children (a
goodly-sized town), are to-day living in our
city in a condition the most destructive to
health, happiness, and morals that could possibly be devised. As you look into these abodes
of wretchedness, filth and disease, the inmates
manifest the same lethargic habits as animals,
burrowing in the ground. They are, indeed,
half narcotized by the constant inhalation of the
emanations of their own bodies, and by a prolonged absence of light and fresh air. Here we
never find sound health, while the constant sickness rate ranges from 75 to 90 per cent.

NOW, as to the second condition under which
we find the laboring classes. It is estimated
by the police that the tenant-house population of New York reaches the enormous figure
of 500,000 or about half of the
Tenant-House total number of inhabitants.
Population The great and striking fact in
regard to the domiciliary
condition of the tenant-house class is over-

crowding and deficient sunlight and fresh air.
The landlord of the poor tenant-house has two
principal motives — first, to pack as many people as he can in a given space, and second, to
make as few improvements and repairs as possible.

The tenant-houses are of two classes, viz.,
the front and the rear. The latter is closely

Third Avenue.

FRONT			No. 70.	No. 68.	DWELLINGS.	
No. 98	98 Rear.	Yard.	70 Rear.	68 Rear.	Stable. 22	No. 22
No. 96						No. 20

Twelfth Stree. — Eleventh Stree.

PLAN SHOWING REAR TENANT-HOUSES, NEAR A STABLE,
IN THE SEVENTEENTH WARD, 1865

allied to the cellar; being shut out from air and
sunlight, it is generally damp, gloomy, and
filthy. The space between the front and rear
house, familiarly called the "well hole," contains the privy and cesspool, the emanations
from which are closely confined to this space,
and slowly but constantly prevade with their
disgusting odors all the rooms and recesses.

The tenant-house has frequently been described by sensation writers, with all its miseries, its diseases and its deaths. But no pen nor pencil can sketch the living reality. It is only by personal inspection that one can learn to what depths of social and physical degradation human beings can descend. Said a committee appointed by your body to investigate the condition of the tenant-houses of New York:

"Sitting together upon the same broken box, lying together upon the same dirty straw, covered by the same filthy shreds, vieing with each other in the utterance of foul obscenities, you have a picture of the mass of corruption and squalid misery gathered inside the walls of that unventilated building in Mission Place. In that single house there was that which made the soul sicken and turn in horror from the sight. Vice, with its pretentious brow, and wretchedness, with hollow cheek and sunken, glazed eye, were there; hunger and lust stood side by side, petit larceny and cold-blooded murder were holding converse."

THE inspectors describe more or less minutely a large number of tenant-houses, and also of groups:

" 'Cat Alley' is the local designation of a group of dilapidated tenant-houses in an alley on Cannon Street. The alley is unpaved, and is excessively filthy. The privy is a small and broken-down structure, covering only a part of

the vault, which is now full almost to overflowing. The inhabitants are degraded, both
Cat physically and socially. In several of
Alley the domiciles, at the time of our last inspection, there was neither bedstead nor
table. Twelve of these families were found in a
wretched condition, and all the children we saw
were covered with dirt, and presented the in-
tensest aspects of scrofulous disease; their sore
eyes, encrusted heads, and dehumanizing appearance, told the story of want and neglect, and
of greater evils to come.

"Five small houses, two and a half stories in
height, including the basements, each containing apartments for six families, front on an alley
called Rivington Place. This alley is always in
a filthy condition. The houses on it are small
and overcrowded. The 30 families that reside
in these five houses have no other water supply
than that which two hydrants furnish in the exterior courtyard; while for this population of
nearly 200 persons, of all ages, there are but two
privy vaults, and, at the time of the last inspection of the quarters, these vaults were filled
nearly to the surface. In the year 1849, 42 individuals died here in three weeks of cholera,
and not one recovered that was taken sick. The
reasons are plain: they have no ventilation, and
the houses being double, the exhalations from
one apartment are inhaled by the other.

"At No. — West Twenty-fifth Street, a

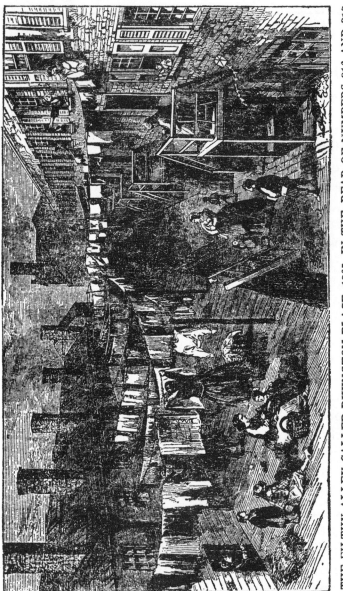

THE FILTHY ALLEY CALLED RIVINGTON PLACE, 1865, IN THE REAR OF NUMBERS 316 AND 318 RIVINGTON STREET

wretched tenement of two apartments, the rooms occupied by one familty. The sitting-room is about 10x12 feet, and the bedroom about 5x12, without a single window or air hole. These rooms were occupied in the hot month of July by a colored female, having pulmonary consumption, and her two children. Here she died, shortly after we made the inspection of her domicilium; having no money nor friends, a Christian burial was denied her for four days, although the neighbors acquainted the police of the fact, and they the Health Warden."

"RAG PICKERS ROW" is thus described: "The houses are of wood, two stories, with attic and basement. The attic rooms are used to deposit the filthy rags and bones as they are taken from gutters and slaughter-houses. The yards are filled with

Rag Pickers Row

dirty rags hung up to dry, send-ing forth their stench to all the neighborhood, and are exceed-ingly nauseous, operating upon me as an emetic. The tenants are all Germans of the lowest order, having no national nor personal pride; they are exceedingly filthy in person, and their bed-clothes are as dirty as the floors they walk on; their food is of the poorest quality, and their feet and heads, and doubtless their whole bodies, are anasarcous, suffering from what they call rheumatism, but which is in reality a prostrate nervous system, the result of foul air air and inadequate supply of nutritious food. They have a peculiar taste for the association of dogs and cats, there being about 50 of the former and 30 of the latter. The whole number of apartments is 32, occupied by 28 families, number 120 in all, 60 adults and 60 children. The yards are all small, and the sinks running over with filth."

S AYS a visitor in the Eighth Ward: "The instances are many in which one or more families, of from three to seven or more members, of all ages and both sexes, are congregated in a single and often contracted apartment. Here they eat, drink, *Tenant-House* sleep, work, dress and undress, *Degeneration* without the possibility of that privacy which an innate modesty imperatively demands. In sickness and in health it is the same.

"What is the consequence? The sense of shame — the greatest, surest safeguard of virtue, except the grace of God — is gradually blunted, ruined, and finally destroyed. New scenes are witnessed and participated in, with a countenance of brass, the very thought of which, once, would have filled the sensitive heart of modesty with pain, ad covered its cheek with burning blushes. The mind of one thus brought in daily and nightly contact with such

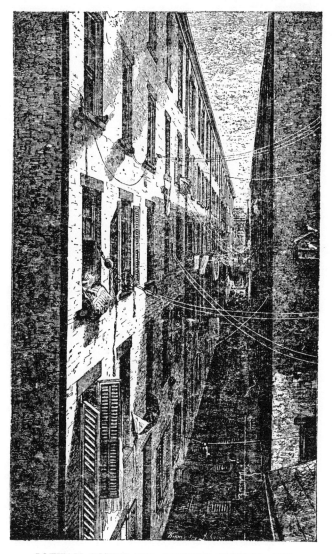

GOTHAM COURT, ON CHERRY STREET, 1865

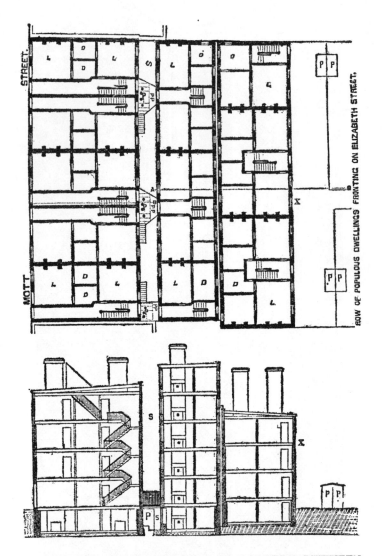

TRANSVERSE SECTIONAL VIEW OF ROOKERY BETWEEN
BROADWAY AND BOWERY, 1865

In its dark, damp cellar, 18 feet square by 7 high, lived 7 persons

L, LIVING ROOM; D, DORMITORY

scenes must become greatly debased, and its fall, before the assaults of vice, rendered almost certain."

Another writes: "These houses seem to be always open to newcomers, and, in some way or other, they can accommodate them. I have found three families, of men, women, and children, in one room; there they lived and there they slept. Can any one doubt that there must be a rapid declension of morals in both parents and children, or that a bar is here opposed to moral and religious instruction, or that this state of things is consequent on the circumstances and condition of life?"

I could give you many details of other tenant-houses, the reputation of which is a reproach to any city in the civilized world. Such is "Gotham Court," "Rotten Row," "The Great Eastern," "Sebastopol," "Quality Row," "Bummer's Retreat," etc. Speaking of the tenant-house, the Rev. Dr. Muhlenburg says:

" 'Their homes!' that cold and damp cellar, about as tenantable as your coal vault! Do you call that a home for the distressed body, crowded in one corner there, swollen with the pains of rheumatism? Or that close apartment, heated or stifling in preparing the evening meal, on the shattered stove — that suffocating room, where you would not stop within for a moment — is that the home which you think so favorable for the worn asthmatic, catching every

breath as if the last?   Ask any clergyman, he
will tell you with how little satisfaction he
makes his visits among the poor, when they are
laboring among disease; how he never has the

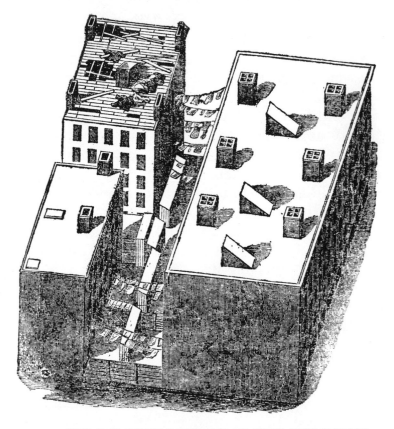

"THE GREAT EASTERN," NUMBER 115 EAST 37TH STREET,
1865

heart to speak of comfort for the soul, when
discomforts of the body call so loudly for re-

lief, and for which the scanty aid he can minister seems akin to mockery!"

M R. N. P. WILLIS who witnessed the "draft"
riots thus truthfully and graphically describes the inmates of tenant-houses:
"The high brick blocks and closely packed
houses where the mobs originated, seemed to
be literally hives of sickness and vice.
The   It was wonderful to see, and difficult to
Rioters   believe, that so much misery, disease
and wretchedness can be huddled together and hidden by high walls, unvisited and
unthought of, so near our own abodes. Lewd,
but pale and sickly young women, scarce decent
in their ragged attire, were impudent and scattered everywhere in the crowd. But what numbers of these poorer classes are deformed —
what numbers are made hideous by self-neglect
and infirmity! Alas! human faces look so
hideous with hope and self-respect all gone!
And female forms and features are made so
frightful by sin, squalor, and debasement! To
walk the streets as we walked them, in those
hours of conflagration and riot, was like wit-
nessing the day of judgment, with every wicked
thing revealed, every sin and sorrow blazingly
glared upon, every hidden abomation laid bare
before hell's expectant fire? The elements of
popular discord are gathered in these wretch-
edly constructed tenement houses, where pov-

erty, disease, and crime find an abode. Here
disease in its most loathsome forms propagates
itself. Unholy passions rule in the domestic
circle. Everything, within and without, tends
to physical and moral degradation."

SUCH, Mr. Chairman, is the external and internal sanitary condition of the homes of
500,000 people in the City of New York to-
day, as revealed by this inspection. It requires
no extraordinary amount of medical knowledge
to determine the physical condi-
Tenant-House   tion of this immense population,
Rot   living under such circumstances.
Even though no devastating
epidemic is found ravaging the tenant-house,
yet the first sight of the wretched inmates con-
vinces you that diseases far more destructive to
health and happiness, because creating no
alarm, are wasting the vital energies, and slowly
but surely consuming the very tissues of the
body.

Here infantile life unfolds its bud, but per-
ishes before its first anniversary. Here youth
is ugly with loathsome diseases and the de-
formities which follow physical degeneracy.
Here the decrepitude of old age is found at
thirty. The poor themselves have a very expressive term for the slow process of decay
which they suffer, viz.: "Tenant-house Rot."
The great majority are, indeed, undergoing a

slow decomposition — a true eremacausis, as the chemists term it. And with this physical degeneration we find mental and moral deterioration. The frequent expression of the poor, "We have no sickness, thank God," is uttered by those whose sunken eyes, pale cheeks, and colorless lips speak more eloquently than words, of the unseen agencies which are sapping the fountains of health. Vice, crime, drunkenness, lust, disease, and death, here hold sway, in spite of the most powerful moral and religious influences.

Religious teachers and Bible readers are beginning to give this class over, as past all remedy, until their physical condition is improved. Their intellects are so blunted and their perceptions so perverted by the noxious atmosphere which they breathe, and the all-pervading filth in which they live, move, and have their being, that they are not susceptible to moral or religious influences. In London, some of the city missionaries have entirely abandoned the tenant-house class. There is, undoubtedly, a depraved physical condition which explains the moral deterioration of these people, and which can never be overcome until we surround them with the conditions of sound health. A child growing up in this pestilential atmosphere becomes vicious and brutal, not from any natural depravity, but because it is mentally incapable of the perceptions of truth.

Most truly does the Inspector of the Fourth
Ward say:

"THERE is a tenant-house cachexy well-
known to such medical men as have a
practical acquaintance with these abodes;
nor does it affect alone the physical condition
of their inmates. It has its moral prototype in
                       an ochlesis of vice — a conta-
Tenant-House   gious   depravity,   to   whose
  Cachexy   malign influence the youthful
                       survivors of the terrible phys-
ical evils to which their infancy is exposed, are
sure to succumb. We often find in persons of
less than middle age, who have long occupied
such confined and filthy premises, a morbid condition of the system unknown elsewhere. The
eye becomes bleared, the senses blunted, the
limbs shrunken and tremulous, the secretions
excedingly offensive. There is a state of pre-
mature decay.

"In this condition of life the ties of nature
seem to be unloosed. Maternal instinct and filial
affection seem to participate in the general decay of soul and body. A kind Providence, whose
hand is visible even here, mercifully provides
that the almost inevitable decay and death
which man's criminal neglect entails on the off-
spring of the unfortunate who dwell in these
dreary mansions, shall elicit comparatively
feeble pangs of parental anguish. To the phys-

ical and moral degradation, the blight of these miserable abodes, where decay reigns supreme over habitation and inhabitant alike, may be plainly traced much of the immorality and crime which prevail among us. The established truth, that, as the corporeal frame deteriorates, man's spiritual nature is liable also to degenerate, receives its apt illustration here."

B UT, sir, acute diseases, and those frequently of the most destructive character, prevail at all seasons among the tenant-house population, and generally with fearful fatality. Although the last summer and autumn were unusually healthy, these records show *Prevailing* the prevalence of a vast amount *Diseases* of diseases among the poor of New York. These diseases are of a kind that always originate in or are aggravated by the crowding of families in unventilated apartments, want of sunlight and pure air, house and street filth, etc.

First Ward: The diseases prevalent in this district the past season have been principally typhus, measles, diarrhoea, dysentery, cholera morbus, cholera infantum, and marasmus. Diarrhoeal diseases are most prevalent in those insalubrious quarters already described, and at a season when the exciting causes are at their greatest stage of development and activity.

Second and Third Wards: Typhus fever made

its appearance in tenant-houses, and in two or three instances spread through all the families immediately exposed. At one place the disease attacked successively every member of the family immediately exposed, but was prevented from spreading further by free ventilation.

Fifth Ward: The slips, in consequence of receiving the sewerage of the district and surrounding parts of the city, are generally foul and the undoubted source of much sickness. Smallpox has prevailed more extensively than for many years back. Typhus and typhoid fevers have been prevalent over the whole district.

Eighth Ward: The prevailing diseases of the past season have been fevers of the typhus, typhoid, remittent and intermittent types, cholera infantum, scarlatina, dysentery, and diarrhoea, all confined to densely populated tenements. The typhus and typhoid fevers have been of a malignant type in two houses, twelve out of eighteen cases proving fatal.

Ninth Ward: The prevailing diseases during the past season have been typhoid fever, dysentery, diarrhoea, scarlet fever, measles, and a few cases of variola.

SIXTH Ward: The seeds of disease exist everywhere, and although removable and susceptible of sanitary control, they are yet uncontrolled, and at any time may spring into activity and a terrific life, that shall only have the power and effect of death. Cholera, when it visits these shores again, will first break forth here, if proper sanitary measures be neglected. Ty-phus fever nests exist in all parts of the district; and it has been traced from these nests to every ward in the city, spreading the disease not only in the worst localities, but into the homes of the industrious, the wealthy, and the highest classes of society. This disease is now on the increase, and if proper sanitary measures are not adopted to remove the predisposing and the infecting causes, we may again have an epidemic of that scourge.

Seeds of Disease Uncontrolled

Fourteenth Ward: There have been attended in this district, during the last year, over 200 cases of typhoid and typhus fever by one dispensary physician; also, 70 cases of dysentery, and 50 cases of smallpox. There is one particular locality which has contributed to the spread and intensity of the fever contagion, viz.: the little street known as Jersey Street. It is always filthy, and the effluvia arising therefrom is extremely offensive. The privies are generally full nearly to overflowing, and the yards are also in a dirty condition, heaps of refuse matter being allowed to remain and to accumulate continually in many of them. There is no sewer in this little street, though the streets at each end are sewered.

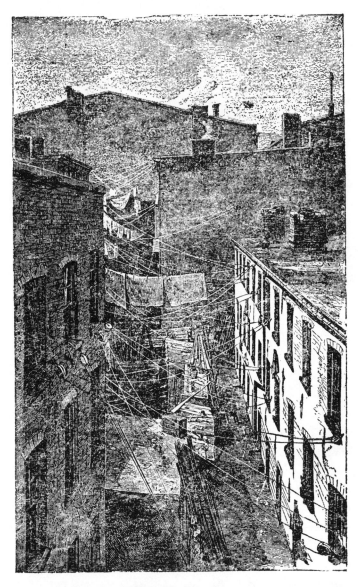

A PERPETUAL FEVER-NEST: REAR TENANT-HOUSES
IN WASHINGTON STREET, 1865

TENTH WARD: The most prominent diseases during the past year have been phthisis, typhoid and scarlet fevers, cholera infantum, dysentery, smallpox, and diphtheria. They were most prevalent in the poorest part of the district, having the *Where Disease* lowest ground, the filthiest *Flourishes* streets, and the most dense population of poor and careless people, who are crowded in the numerous tenant-houses, shanties, and small dwellings, which were built for one or two families, but are now made to contain from five to ten.

Nineteenth Ward: The diseases that have chiefly prevailed during the past season are dysentery, diarrhoea, cholera morbus, cholera infantum and the exanthematous fevers. They were of the most frequent occurrence in the most crowded and insalubrious quarters.

Fifteenth Ward: Since the commencement of the survey, scarlet fever, typhoid fever, smallpox, and cholera infantum have prevailed in the tenant-houses of this ward. Six cases of smallpox occurred in one of three thickly peopled rows of such dwellings, and the disease was communicated to a child in an adjacent street, who had been playing in the infected neighborhood. Seven cases of typhoid also occurred in a court among children, and this was within a few doors of better class houses.

Eleventh Ward: Typhus and typhoid fevers

have been found prevailing in all sections of this district. Smallpox, scarlatina, measles, and pulmonary diseases are met with in almost every street. Typhus is the most typical of the preventable diseases that abound in the Eleventh Ward. Cholera infantum and obstinate diarrhoeal maladies were prevalent in the rear tenements and throughout the lowest streets during the summer and autumn.

To give you an idea of the wide prevalence of these diseases, I will notice one or two more in detail.

SMALLPOX is the very type of preventable diseases. We have a safe and sure preventive in thorough vaccination. And yet this loathsome disease is at this moment an epidemic in New York. In two days' time, the inspectors found 644 cases, and in two weeks, *Smallpox* upward of 1,200; and it was estimated that only about one-half were discovered. In many large tenant-houses, six, eight, and ten cases were found at the same time. They found it under every conceivable condition tending to promote its communicability. It was in the street cars, in the stages, in the hacks, on the ferry-boats, in junk-shops, in cigar-stores, in candy-shops, in the families of tailors and seamstresses, who were making clothing for wholesale stores, in public and in private charities. I hold in my hand a list

of cases of smallpox found existing under circumstances which show how widespread is this
disease. Bedding of a fatal case of smallpox
was sold to a rag-man; case in a room where
candy and daily papers were sold; case on a
ferry-boat; woman was attending bar and acting
as nurse to her husband who had smallpox;
girl was making cigars while scabs were falling
from her skin; seamstress was making shirts
for a Broadway store, one of which was thrown
over the cradle of a child sick of smallpox; tailors making soldiers' clothing, have their children, from whom the scabs were falling,
wrapped in the garments; a woman selling
vegetables had the scabs falling from her face,
among the vegetables, etc., etc. Instances of
this kind can be quoted at any length, but these
examples are sufficient to show that smallpox
spreads uncontrolled throughout our city. And
they show, too, how this disease is disseminated
abroad. Says the Inspector of the Fourth
Ward:

IN localities where smallpox prevailed I
found, in some instances within a few feet
of the patients, tailors at work for our best
clothing establishments. Such infected vest-
ments — worse than the tunic of the Centaur —
bring disease and death not only to the wearers,
but to many others. The occupant of the
crowded tenant-house procures from such a

source a coat or a blanket, and soon a loathsome pest attacks the
Smallpox in Tailored   young and unprotected
Garments   members of his family,
and ultimately spreads
through the entire quarter, destroying life after
life and endangering the health of a whole community.

"Smallpox, suddenly breaking out in some
secluded rural district, often owes its unsuspected origin to the above causes. In the
remote solitude of the ocean the seaman opens
the chest in which he has deposited such obnoxious apparel, and from this Pandora's box
scatters the seeds of pestilence among his com-
rades, which, ripening, shall spread its germs
to distant ports."

Or, what is more striking, take the following
from the report of the Inspector of the Fifth
Ward:

"The largest wholesale establishments for the
sale of dry goods on this side of the Atlantic
Ocean are in immediate contact with the tenant-
houses of the worst class, and which are infested
with smallpox and typhus fever. The two
freight depots and the principal passenger depot
of the Railroad Company are in the same close
association with these nests of infection. In the
region immediately surrounding are also situated several hotels, and a large number of
boarding-houses, whose inmates are thus in dan-

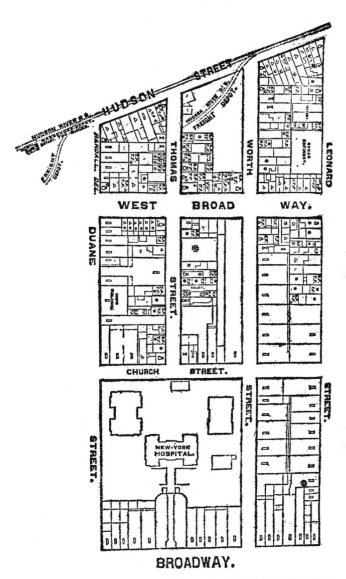

A REGION OF SMALLPOX AND TYPHUS FEVER, 1865

ger of personal contact with these diseases any
moment. West Broadway, running through the
very centre of the district, is traversed by five
different lines of railway cars, with an average
of five cars passing every minute, and carrying
millions of passengers yearly by the very doors
of these houses. Broadway, at but a short distance removed, is the principal thoroughfare of
the city.   Hudson Street on the west is also a
leading route for city travel; and the cross
streets of the district are traversed daily by multitudes to reach various lines of steamboats,
cars, and steamships, which leave the city opposite this point.

"All this large amount of daily travel passes
through a region always containing cases of
typhus fever, and largely infected with smallpox.   Is it any cause of surprise that cases of
these diseases are here contracted, to be carried
to distant sections of the country, there to de-
velop themselves, to the surprise and alarm of
whole neighborhoods?   It is also well to remember that several large livery stables are located
in the immediate neighborhood, whose vehicles,
it is well-known, are frequently employed to
carry persons, suffering from these diseases, to
hospitals, or to attend at funerals.   These vehicles are, perhaps, immediately afterward
driven to the various car and steamboat lines
to secure passengers, who are thus exposed in
the most dangerous manner to these diseases."

SECOND only to smallpox as a preventable disease, but of a more fatal character, is typhus fever. Typhus is greatly aggravated by domestic filth, and by overcrowding, with deficient ventilation. The inspectors found and located by street and num-
Typhus ber no less than 2,000 cases of this
Fever most contagious and fatal disease. Commencing in a large tenant-house in Mulberry Street, it was traced from locality to locality, in the poorer quarters, until it was found to have visited nearly every section of the city. It became localized in many tenant-houses and streets, where it still remains, causing a large amount of sickness and mortality.

At Mulberry Street, in a notoriously filthy house, it has existed for more than four years. This house has a population of about 320, which is renewed every few months. During the period alluded to, there have been no less than 60 deaths by fever in this single house, and 240 cases. To-day this fever is raging uncontrolled in that house, creating more orphans than many well-fought battles. Every new family which enters these infected quarters is sure to fall a victim to this pestilential disease.

The tenant-house No. — East Seventeenth Street, which reaks with filth, gives the same history; upward of 85 cases, with a large percentage of deaths, occurred in this single house during the past season. And still it remained unclean and open to new tenants. I could mention scores of these houses in every part of the tenant-house district where typhus has apparently taken up its abode, and from whence it sends out in every direction its deadly streams.

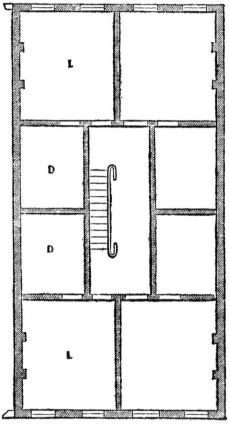

Not only have single houses become centres of contagion, b u t this fever has, in many instances, b e c o m e localized in crowded streets, which today are almost impassable on account of the heaps of garbage, and t h e courts and alleys of which are reeking w i t h f i l t h , making them great centres of pestilence.

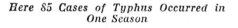

PLAN OF FEVER-NEST, EAST 17TH STREET, 1865

Here 85 Cases of Typhus Occurred in One Season

From many of these tenements whole families have been swept away.

Jersey Street, a short but uncleaned avenue, adjacent to a fashionable part of Broadway, is another great depot of fever, which, according to these records, frequently contained upward

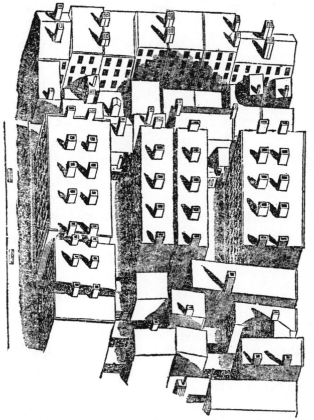

BIRD'S-EYE VIEW OF FEVER-NEST, 1865, NOT FAR
FROM BROADWAY AND FIFTH AVENUE

of thirty cases in progress at one time.   East Eleventh Street, between First and Second Avenues, now, as all the past summer, in a hor-

ribly filthy condition, is a local habitation of fever of the worst type. The same statement may
be made of nearly every district where the
tenant-houses are especially crowded, and the
streets, courts, and alleys are unusually filthy.

I NTESTINAL diseases, as cholera infantum,
diarrhoea, dysentery, typhoid fever, etc.,
which arise from, or are intensely aggravated by the emanations from putrescible material in streets, courts, and alleys, or from cesspools, privies, drain pipes, sewers,
Intestinal   etc., were prevalent in the tenant-
Affections   house districts, creating, as usual,
a vast amount of sickness, and a
large infant mortality. Very generally these
diseases were directly traceable to the decomposing filth, and in some instances were stopped
by the removal of the nuisance.

The Inspector of the Eighth Ward reports:
"Cholera infantum has probably consigned
many more to the grave during the past summer than all other diseases in my inspection
district. In every case examined I have found
it associated with some well-marked course of
insalubrity; vegetable and animal decomposition have been the most prominent causes. That
fifty per cent die from preventable causes in
my inspection district I do not doubt."

The Inspector of the Sixth Ward says: "The
mortality among children is fearfully high,

many families having lost all their children; others four out of five or six."

THE Inspector of the Ninth Ward says he found among the people living near the mouth of an open sewer: "That no less than twenty-nine cases of dysentery and diarrhœa,

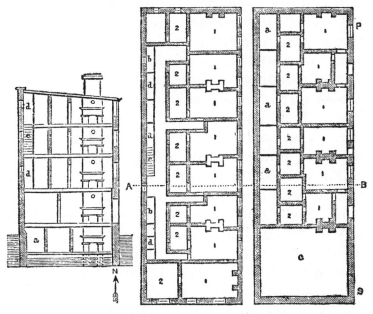

PLAN OF MONROE STREET FEVER-NEST, 1865

five of which had terminated fatally, had occurred during the three weeks immediately preceding his inspection." He adds: "Now, when we take into consideration the fact that there are only twenty-two

Living at a Sewer's Mouth

dwellings on this square (a considerable portion of it being occupied by a large lumber-
yard), and that all these cases had occurred
within a period of about twenty-one days, the
ratio becomes appalling. How many cases
may have occurred subsequently, I have not
sought to ascertain, my time being fully occupied in the inspection of the other parts of my
district. But a still more direct and specific action of the poisonous emanations proceeding
from this obstructed sewerage, manifested itself
in the dwelling on the corner of West and
Gansevoort streets, which is in the closest
proximity to the outlet of the sewer. Here I
learned, upon inquiry, that typhoid fever had
prevailed almost continuously during the preceding winter, and I found three severe cases of
dysentery at the time of my visit."

But I will not occupy time with further details of the evidence which this inspection furnishes of the vast accumulation of the causes of
unhealthiness which exist in New York, and of
the wide prevalence of contagious diseases
arising therefrom or aggravated thereby.

The next point of inquiry is as to the effect
of these conditions upon the public health of
the city. Our constituted health authorities
claim that notwithstanding this excessive concentration of the causes of disease around and
in the homes of half of our population, the
death-rate of New York is very low. To prop-

erly understand this statement, we must inquire what is the rate of death from inevitable causes.

IT has been estimated by careful writers on vital statistics that 17 in 1,000 living persons annually die from inevitable causes. That is, in a community of 1,000 persons living under circumstances such that persons die only from old age, cancer, casualties, etc.,

The Normal Death-Rate 17 will die annually, and no more. And this number is the maximum that will die without the occurrence of some disease due to a removable cause. Taking this standard as the absolute necessary death-rate, we can readily estimate the number of unnecessary or preventable deaths which occur in any community.

Says the Registrar-General of England (Twentieth Annual Report): "Any deaths in a people exceeding 17 in 1,000 annually are unnatural deaths. If the people were shot, drowned, burnt, poisoned by strychnine, their deaths would not be more unnatural than the deaths wrought clandestinely by diseases in excess of the quota of natural death — that is, in excess of seventeen in 1,000 living."

TAKING this as the standard, let us see how the death-rate of New York compares with it. It is claimed by the city officials that notwithstanding the vast accumulation of the uni-

versally-recognized causes of disease, New York
has a low death-rate.   It is not
Death-Rate of   reasonable   to   suppose   this
New York   statement true, nor is it true, as
will presently appear.   It is
stated very truly in the City Inspector's Report
for 1863, that "it is only by taking a connected
view of a period of years that a correct judgment can be formed of the state of health of a
city," and upon this basis let us determine what
is the mortality of New York.

Take the 11 years preceding the last census,
viz., 1860, excluding, however, 1854, the year of
the cholera.   I select this period because it includes the three last census returns, and it is
only where we have the census returns with the
mortality records that we have accurate data for
our estimates.   Now, the City Inspector's own
records (reports of 1863, page 192) show that
during the period referred to, the death-rate of
New York City was never below 28 in the 1,000,
and twice exceeded 40 in the 1,000, the average
being as high as 33 in the 1,000.   These deductions are made directly from the City Inspector's
Reports, and, as they are claimed to be infal-
lible, these conclusions cannot be controverted.

Now, when you remember that the highest
death-rate fixed by sanitary writers for inevitable deaths is 17 in 1,000, and that all deaths
above that standard are considered preventable,
it is apparent what a fearful sacrifice of life

there is in New York. Estimated at the very
minimum death-rate of the last decennial period, viz.: 28 in 1,000, New York annually lost
11 from preventable deaths in 1,000 of her population, or upwords of 7,000 yearly, on an average, giving the enormous sum total for this
period of 77,000 preventable deaths.

It may be urged that cities never can attain
to this standard of healthfulness, but English
writers maintain that the rate of 17 in the 1,000
is the true measure of the public health, and
that even the most populous towns may yet be
brought up to it. Nor can we doubt that there
is much plausibility in the assertion, when we
find the mortality in Philadelphia fall to 18 in
1,000 , and that of London gradually descend
from 30 in 1,000 to 22 in 1,000.

IT is maintained, also, that New York has a
lower death-rate than London or Philadelphia. Let us see how far this assertion is
sustained by the records of the health authorities of those cities. During the decennial period
preceding, but includ-
New York, London, and ing 1860, and exclud-
Liverpool Compared ing 1854, as in the
former comparison,
the minimum mortality in London was 20 in
1,000, the maximum 24 in 1,000, the mean
about 22 in 1,000. These figures are from the
Registrar-General Reports.

The rate of mortality of Philadelphia for the same period was as follows: Minimum 18 in 1,000, maximum 23 in 1,000, mean about 20 in 1,000. These figures are from the report of Dr. Jewell, long the able Health Officer of that city. Placed in their proper relation, these mortality statistics read as follows: The number of deaths to the 1,000 living for the ten years, 1850—60 inclusive, but exclusive of 1854, is for

	Min.	Max.	Av.
London	20	24	22
Philadelphia	18	23	20
New York	28	41	33

If, then, New York had as low an average death-rate as Philadelphia, she would have saved 13 in 1,000 of her population during that period, or in 1860, 10,577. These figures may seem excessive, but they are careful deductions from the annual returns of the several cities. And yet it is reiterated year after year by the City Inspector, that "New York City, at this day, can lay claim to the privilege of being numbered with the most healthy in the world."

With what consummate justice did Dr. Jewell administer this withering rebuke to our pretentious official. "It is unnecessary," he says, in his report of 1860, "to comment upon this extraordinary statement, when the above figures contradict so positively the assertion. It is to be regretted that the inspector had not availed himself of the above statistical information, which would have obliged him to have presented a widely different statement, although one indicating a more severe pressure of sanitary evils, upon the health of their population, than his report develops."

BUT excessive as is this death-rate, it is not the full measure of the penalty which we pay to the demon of filth. A high death-rate from the diseases which it engenders or intensifies, always implies a large amount of sickness. It is estimated by competent *Constant* authority that there are 28 cases of *Sickness* sickness for every death. On this basis of estimate what an enormous amount of unnecessary sickness exists in our midst! Nor is this a mere supposition. I have an accurate census of many groups of families of that portion of our population who live immured in filth, and here we find the constant sickness-rate excessive. It is no uncommon thing to find it 50, 60, and 70 per cent.

I WISH now to call your attention to the fact that great as is our mortality and sickness rate, its excess is not equally distributed over the entire population, but falls exclusively upon the poor and helpless. One-half, at least, of the population of New York have a death-rate no higher than the people of a healthy country

town, while the death pressure upon the other
half is frightfully
Where the Death Pressure   severe. For ex-
Is Greatest   ample, the Seventeenth   W a r d,
which is inhabited principally by the wealthy
class and has but few tenant-houses, has a death-
rate of but 17 in 1,000, or only the death-rate
from inevitable causes; but the Sixth and
Fourth Wards, which are occupied by the laboring classes, have a death-rate varying from
36 to 40 in 1,000.

Thus it appears that while the average death-
rate of the city is very high, it is principally
sustained by those Wards where the tenant-
house population is the most numerous. We
find this excess of mortality just where we found
the causes of diseases existing most numerously.
And when we sift the matter further, we find
that the excess of mortality is not even equally
distributed over these populous poor Wards, but
is concentrated upon individual tenant-houses.
For example, while the mortality of the Sixth
Ward is nearly 40 in 1,000, the mortality of its
large tenant-houses is as high as 60 to 70 in
1,000. The following is a recent census of a
large but not exceptional tenant-house of that
Ward: Number of families in the house, 74;
persons, 349; deaths, 18, or 53 in 1,000; constant
sickness, 1 in 3; deaths of children, 1 in 6, or at
the rate of 16 in 1,000.

The following table illustrates the distribution of the mortality of New York among the different classes of inhabitants at the last census:

Average mortality of entire
city .... 28 in 1,000
Mortality of better class..... 10 to 17 "   "
Mortality of tenant-house.... 50 " 60 "   "

BUT I should not do justice to this branch of inquiry without noticing the alleged causes of the high mortality of New York. The first is the large foreign immigration. The reliance to be placed upon that scapegoat may be readily shown. Em-

Some Scapegoats— igration occurs to this
Foreign Immigration country under two conditions: 1. The emigrant is driven from home by famine, in which case the poorer class emigrate, or, 2, he is allured by advantages for labor or business, when the middle classes principally emigrate.

Now, it is under the latter circumstancees that emigration generally takes place to the United States. This is seen in the vast sums of money which the emigrants now annually bring, and the amounts which they return to their friends as the result of their labor. This class is always very hardy and healthy, as is proved by the small mortality that occurs *in transitu* being but 4.31 per cent for ten years. Besides, we have the official statements of the Commissioners of Emigration that but 3 per cent remain in the city.

But the City Inspector himself shows the utter fallacy of this alleged cause of excessive mortality in his report for 1860, in which he makes the true explanation, and attributes to its proper

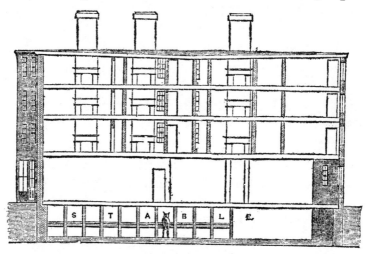

A SIXTH WARD FEVER-NEST WITH DEATH-RATE
OF 53 IN 1,000

cause whatever increased mortality arises from emigrants. He says:

"Most of the children who arrive in this city from foreign ports, although suffering from the effects of a protracted voyage, bad accommodations, and worse fare, do not bring with them any marked disease beyond those which, with proper care, nursing, and wholesome air, could not be easily overcome. The causes of this excessive mortality must be searched for in this

city, and are readily traceable to the wretched
habitations in which parents and children are
forced to take up their abode; in the contracted
alleys, the tenement house, with its hundreds of
occupants, where each cooks, eats, and sleeps in
a single room, without light or ventilation, surrounded with filth, an atmosphere foul, fetid,
and deadly, with none to console with or advise
them, or to apply to for relief when disease
invades them."

AGAIN, it is alleged that the floating population causes the excess of deaths. But it
has been established by Dr. Playfair that
the floating population is the most healthy.
The same is true of wandering tribes, of a moving army, and equally of in-
The Floating dividuals. But when they fix
Population their habitations or encamp,
that moment the causes of dis-
ease begin to gather about them, and unless sanitary regulations are carefully observed, diseases, such as fever, diarrhoeal affections, etc.,
begin to prevail.

The poor population of New York is to-day
but an immense army in camp, upon small
territory, crowded into old filthy dwellings, and
without the slightest police regulation for cleanliness. If this army should abandon its camp
and begin a roving life in the country, all the
diseases now prevalent would disappear. And

it must be added, that if these deserted and uncleaned tenements should immediately be filled
by healthy people from the country, the new
tenants would at once begin to suffer from all
the pestilential diseases now indigenous to that
part of the city.

I have now laid before you, as briefly as possible, the accumulated evidence that New York
is to-day full to repletion with all the causes
which originate and intensify the most loathsome and fatal diseases known to mankind.

This evidence proves that at least half a million of its population are literally submerged
in filth, and half-stifled in an atmosphere
charged with all the elements of death. I have
demonstrated that the legitimate fruits of her
sanitary evils is an excessively high death-rate
and a correspondingly large sickness rate.

THE all-important question which now concerns us as citizens, and you as practical
legislators, is, can these evils be remedied?
We answer, yes. In the first place the
streets can be kept clean. Other cities
accomplish t h i s
Can the Causes of Disease object, and there-
Be Removed? fore New York can,
and we have strik-
ing illustrative examples. In certain portions
of the city the streets are as clean as this
floor. They are swept daily, and scarcely a

particle of dust is left in the streets or gutters the year round. But they are cleaned by private contract of the people residing upon them. What individual enterprise can do for whole squares, surely a corporation so lavish in money as New York ought to be able to do for the city at large.

The courts, alleys, cesspools, and privies can be cleansed and kept in good condition. There are tenant-houses which are as clean in all their alleys, courts, and cellars as the best-kept private houses. These are dwellings for the poor in which the landlord takes especial interest. What is done for the surroundings of one of these houses, may be done for all. But the tenant-houses of the worst class may be quickly placed in a good sanitary condition.

THE inspectors furnish many examples of this fact. They were frequently mistaken in their inspection for an official, and when their visit to the tenant-houses was reported to the landlord, he hastened to renovate the building. Some of the most *Improvements During* filthy quarters were so *the Inspection* completely changed within f o r t y - e i g h t hours that the inspectors could scarcely recognize the locality. The Inspector of the Eighth Ward says:

"The sanitary improvement in my district

during the progress of my inspection was plainly visible. Exceedingly filthy places, overflowing cesspools, and privies, which were numerous in my first visit, were suddenly cleaned. Often upon my second visit, with paper and pencil in my hand to sketch the filthy scene, I would find the quarters cleaned and whitewashed, and the air, instead of being laden with disagreeable odors, would be comparatively pure and wholesome. Many of these sudden transitions were from fear of the presumption that my inspection had some official authority; but

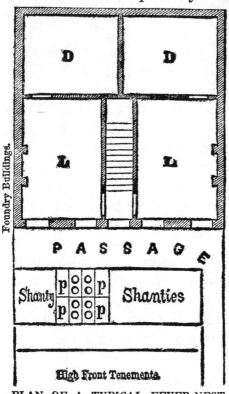

PLAN OF A TYPICAL FEVER-NEST, 1865

the greater part were brought about by explaining to the people the necessity of cleanliness.

"Pools of filthy water from obstructions at the street corners, and accumulated along the gut-

ters, would quickly disappear, when the people
would be convinced of the deleterious effect
upon the public health. It will be well for the
inhabitants of New York City, and especially
for those of this section, when there shall be
laws not only to compel them to keep their
houses and surroundings clean and free from
the effluvia resulting from vegetable and animal
decomposition, but to prevent the overcrowding of tenant-houses, where fatal diseases are
generated, and where death walks around."

THE tenant-house population is susceptible of
infinite improvement, when once rescued
from the reign of filth, and restored to a
pure atmosphere and clean homes. The poor
live in these wretched tenements because they
are compelled to, and not
How to Improve   from choice. They uni-
the People   versally complain that they
cannot escape from domes-
tic and street filth. It surrounds and pervades
their habitations, always accumulating, and
never diminishing. The most tidy house-wife,
compelled to live in the midst of this ocean of
rubbish, with all its degrading associations, soon
finds the same level, and from this she can be
rescued only by giving her again a clean and
well-ordered home. And such a home every
municipal government is bound tò secure to the
poorest and humblest citizen.

Let the landlord be compelled to keep his house in good repair, supply it with an abundance of pure water, connect the privy with the sewer, open free ventilation, afford means for removal of garbage, and then keep a careful oversight of his tenants, enforcing cleanliness. If this were done, the tenant-house people would immediately improve, and the death-rate, if we may judge from other cities, would fall one-fourth.

Again, the cellar population can be removed from their subterranean abodes, and placed in better homes. Liverpool has solved this problem for us.

In 1847 that city had a cellar population of 20,000; an ordinance was passed forbidding the occupation of underground rooms as residences, with certain restrictions, and within three years the great mass of people in these subterranean haunts were removed to better tenements, with a great reduction of the mortality of the city.

That city, formerly the most unhealthy in England, has continued the reforms thus inaugurated by compelling landlords to improve their tenant-houses, and the result is that it has become one of the healthiest towns of Europe. London has recently taken similar action in regard to cellar tenements. What these cities have done, New York can and ought to do for her public health.

WHAT the diseases which prevail with such fatality in the uncleaned tenant-houses are for the most part preventable, we have the most undoubted evidence. That smallpox is preventable is known to every school-boy, and yet that loathsome disease to-day prevails throughout all the tenant-house districts of New York, without the slightest restraint on the part of our local authorities. Typhus is to-day ravaging the homes of the poor without "let or hindrance," and yet cleanliness and pure air are sure preventives. Of this truth these reports furnish many examples.

A Town That Was Immune

The fever-nest — West Thirty-third Street — is one of a row of tenant-houses five stories high, and contains 16 families. It was in a filthy condition, without Croton water, waste-pipes stopped, sinks overflowing and emitting offensive odors; fever had prevailed all winter, nearly every person in the house having had an attack, four having died. It was never inspected by a city official. The owner was induced to clean the house, and from that date not a case of fever has occurred. The inspector who reports this case very justly adds: "If, when the first case of fever occurred in this building, the owner had been compelled to put it in a good sanitary condition, six human lives would undoubtedly have been saved, besides a great amount of sickness."

Cholera infantum and diarrhoeal affections
are found in their greatest intensity where
putrescible animal matter and domestic filth

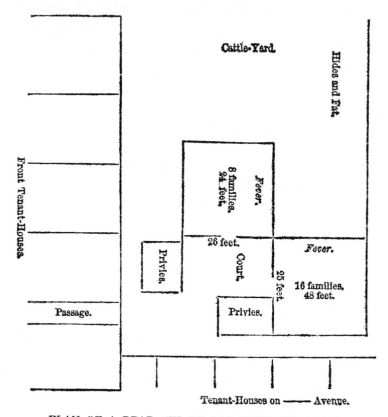

PLAN OF A REAR CUL-DE-SAC FEVER-NEST, 1865

exist. Remove these causes, or remove the patients from the neighborhood, and these diseases generally disappear at once. Diphtheria
is found to be most intense in the vicinity of
unclean stables. It is, therefore, with great

propriety, that the entire class of zymotic diseases are now called "filth and foul air" diseases by the English sanitary writers. Remove
the filth and foul air, and these diseases disappear as effect follows cause.

BUT while it is admitted that the streets of a
town may be cleaned, the condition of the
poor improved, and diseases, under the
most favorable circumstances, prevented, it may
be doubted whether the sanitary condition of
populous towns can be
Can Populous Towns   materially changed, and
Be Improved?   the death-rate greatly
reduced. Yet in Eng-
land, where sanitary science is enthusiastically
cultivated, there is not only no doubt that large
towns can be thus improved, but that the mortality of London itself may be no greater than
that of the country.

Already, indeed, the London *Times* boasts
"that the average of health throughout the City
of London is higher than the average of health
throughout all England, taking town and country together. The mortality in all England is
at the rate of 22.8 in every 1,000 of the population; in the City of London it is at the rate of
22.3 for every 1,000 inhabitants! The improvement has been progressive; it has been slow,
but steady and sure. Gradually the mortality
has decreased, until the yearly death roll of

3,763 has been reduced to 2,904 within a period
of nine years, during which the city has been
under the rule of the Sanitary Commission.
The deaths this year — 22.3 per 1,000, or one in
every forty-five of the inhabitants — are nine
per cent below the general average, and represent a saving of 286 lives. And secondly, this
gratifying result has been obtained in the face
of obstacles which seemed to be almost insur-
mountable."

Liverpool affords a striking example of the
power of sanitary measures, rigidly enforced to
improve the public health. It was formerly the
most unhealthy city of England, being the very
home of typhus, smallpox, and allied preventable diseases. But it adopted vigorous measures of reform, improving its poorer districts,
and the death-rate has fallen eight in 1,000.
Macclesfield, Salisbury, and many other English towns have had their mortality reduced 8,
10, and 15 in 1,000 by the vigorous prosecution
of sanitary improvements. All the populous
towns of that country are moving in this reform,
and, as a result, the general death-rate of towns
is approximating that of the country.

THE Health Officer of London announced that
cleanliness would preserve a town from the
visitations of epidemics. But there must be
cleanliness of the streets, cleanliness of the
courts. cleanliness of the apartments. and clean-

liness of the person.   On the approach of the
cholera in 1849 the
Cleanliness Preserves   town of Worcester,
from Epidemics   England, determined
to test the theory, and
set vigorously to work and cleaned the town
thoroughly, removing everything of an offensive
nature, and adopting the most stringent regulations against the accumulation of filth about or
within the homes of the people.   The result
was that this "destroyer" of unclean cities
made a Passover with the people of Worcester,
for on every lintel and door-post was written
— Cleanliness, Cleanliness.   Not a house was
entered, and the town was saved in the midst
of the most frightful desolation.

New Orleans is another striking example of
the value of civic cleanliness.   Since, by military
regulations, it is kept constantly in a cleanly
condition, it has had no visitation of its old enemy, yellow fever.

The degree of public health of a town is
therefore measured by its cleanliness, and its
capacity for health depends upon its capacity
for cleanliness.

THERE is scarcely a city which has such absolute need of an efficient and intelligent
sanitary government as New York.   On its
small territory three, four, or five millions of
people are yet to be accommodated with houses.

Already there are crowded upon less than eight
of its t h i r t y - t w o
Importance of Sanitary   square miles all of our
Government   commercial, business,
and manufacturing
interests, and the houses of nearly 1,000,000 of
people. And in the natural relations of the poor
and rich, the former consisting of more than
half of the entire population, are crowded into
less than a fourth of this area. Of what vast
importance is it that a wise and intelligent
authority be vigilantly exercised, so that in its
future growth and expansion every condition
pertaining to health shall be secured to its inhabitants!

It is universally conceded that New York has
in the highest degree all the natural advantages of salubrity. Its climate is the mean between the extremes of heat and cold; its topographical peculiarities are admirably adapted
for drainage and sewerage; its exposure is
southern; its shores are swept by two rivers,
which bear seaward everything that enters them
beyond the power of the flowing tide to return
it; its rural surroundings are of the most health-
ful. In every respect it is regarded by competent observers as most favorably located for
cleanliness, and the highest degree of public
health. And there can be no doubt, that should
New York be placed under a wise sanitary government, which would improve all its natural

advantages for health, it would become the
cleanest and healthiest city in the world, and
one of the most delightful places of residence.

BUT this is not a matter which concerns the
citizens of New York alone. The people of
the State have a vital interest in the public
health of our city. Connected as it is by means

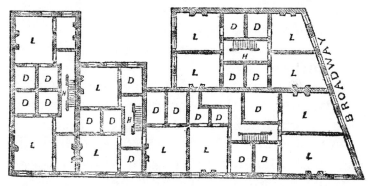

FLOOR-PLAN OF A NEW FEVER-BREEDING STRUCTURE
NEAR BROADWAY AND CENTRAL PARK, 1865

of rapid inter-communication with all parts of
the country, there is every
The Entire Country facility offered for the
Concerned wide diffusion of the
seeds of contagion. It is
estimated by accurate statisticians that no less
than 250,000 persons pass in and out of New
York daily over the ferries and railroads. It
could not fail to happen that if any contagious
disease prevailed in this city, it would be
carried into the country and widely dissem-

inated. And such is now a matter of daily occurrence. There is no doubt that nearly all the
epidemics of smallpox in country towns, and
much of the typhus and similar diseases, have
their origin in New York. I have in my hand
letters from all parts of the State confirming this
statement. They strikingly illustrate the want
of a good sanitary police in New York, and the
power of a great commercial centre to scatter
disease broadcast over the country.

A few of these cases will abundantly illustrate
the point:

Dr. J. S. Sprague, of Cooperstown, Otsego
County, reports the occurrence of twenty-six
cases of smallpox in that town, communicated
by one person in October, 1860, who took the
disease at a hotel in our city, in which a person
with the disease had recently died. He was a
merchant, and came to the city on business.

Dr. C. C. F. Gay, of Buffalo, reports the case
of a female, who arrived from New York in
November, 1860, and was removed from the
cars of the Erie Railroad to the State Line Road,
and proceeded westward. As was afterward ascertained, she had smallpox, and communicated the disease at Columbus, Ohio, where
there were three deaths produced by it. Four
deaths were directly traceable to this exposure,
viz.: three milkmen and one baggage man, all of
whom came in contact with the sick woman.

W. T. Babbitt mentions the case of a young

man who took the disease in this city at a hotel where it was prevailing, at which he stopped while on a visit here, in whom the disease appeared after his return to Olean, in Cattaraugus County.

Dr. M. Jarvis, of Canestota, Madison County, relates the case of a man who visited this city with horses for sale, and was attacked with symptoms of smallpox some ten days after his return to Smithfield, in that county, who communicated the disease to his family, from whom it spread to others in that and, also, in a neighboring town.

DR. C. M. NOBLE, of Waverley, Delaware County, mentions the case of a merchant of that place, who came to this city with his wife, and went to one of our most frequented hotels. Being very much fatigued, they retired to the room provided *Smallpox in a* for them without any particular *Hotel Bedroom* ticular examination of it — but found in the morning that they had been put in a room from which a patient with smallpox had just been removed, without its having been cleansed. The gentleman was seized with a malignant form of that disease after his return home. Two deaths and six cases of smallpox and varioloid resulted from this case.

Dr. S. W. Turner, of Chester, Connecticut,

gives also two cases, one of smallpox and one of varioloid, in that and a neighboring place, which could be traced to this city.

Dr. Snow, the vigilant Health Officer of Providence, R. I., states that smallpox is rarely known in that city, except when imported from New York.

I COULD repeat these details until it was shown that nearly every town in the State, and nearly every city in the country, has been inoculated by New York with this most loathsome disease. The most striking and most melancholy instances of *New York Inoculates* the free dissemination *the Nation* of contagion are found in the army, where whole regiments have been stricken with smallpox through infected clothing manufactured at the homes of the poor, where the disease was prevailing. But these are facts too well known to every medical man, and even to the community, to require further illustration.

What terror smallpox creates in country towns when it attacks its first victim, you very well know. The house where it occurs is quarantined, and not unfrequently the sufferer is deserted by his friends, and left to recover or die, as the case may be. Business with the country is often suspended by the placards posted upon the highways, with the terrifying word "Small-

pox" upon them, and a finger pointing om-
inously to the town. In nine cases out of ten,
another finger should point toward New York,
as the source of the pestilence.

It has been estimated by a competent observer, that every case of smallpox in a country
town costs, by derangement of business alone,
more money than is annually expended upon
its public schools. If we add to this pecuniary
loss the feverish excitement and popular apprehension, and the sufferings and probable death
of the victim from want of proper care, we may
but indifferently estimate the cost to the country
of the prevalence of this disease.

Now, this diffusion of contagion from New
York, we contend, is unnecessary. Every well-
informed medical man knows that we may have
a sanitary police so vigilant, so efficient and so
powerful, that it will not only preserve the public health, but prevent the spread of disease
therefrom. We hold, therefore, that you are not
only called upon to protect the people of the
City of New York from contagious disease, but
equally that you are bound to protect the people of the State from dissemination of pestilence
by every legislative safeguard which sanitary
science can suggest.

THE Sanitary Committee of the Board of
Health, during the prevalence of cholera in
1849, remark in their report:

"The labors of your committee, during the past appalling season of sickness and death, and the awful scenes of *Inefficiency of* degradation, misery, and *Health Organizations* filth developed to them by t h e i r researches, have brought into full view the fact that we have no sanitary police worthy of the name; that we are unprotected by that watchful regard over the public health which common sense dictates to be necessary for the security of our lives, the maintenance of the city's reputation, and the preservation of the interests of the inhabitants."

THIS is a perfectly truthful statement of the present condition of New York. Practically, it is a city without any sanitary government. In its growth it is developing the natural history of a city that utterly ignores all rules and regulations which tend to *Without Sanitary* make the homes of its peo- *Government* ple pleasant and healthy. It is the only city in the civilized world which disregards the Platonic idea that in a model republic medical men should be selected to preserve and promote the public health. Its board of health, the mayor and common council, is an unwieldly body. Its commisioners of health have limited powers, and are equally incompetent.

THE City Inspector's department, which alone
has the machinery for sanitary inspection
and surveillance, is a gigantic imposture. Of
its forty-four health wardens, whose duty it
should be to make house-to-house inspections,
searching out the cause
The City Inspector's   of disease, and using
Department   every known agency for
the control and suppres-
sion of epidemics, many are liquor dealers, and
all are grossly ignorant. Not one has any
knowledge of medical subjects, nor dare they
freely visit such diseases as smallpox, typhus,
or cholera.

During this entire voluntary inspection, extending over six months, health wardens have
rarely been known to visit infected quarters, although smallpox, fever, etc., etc., have been prevalent, and the city has been in a most disgrace-
fully filthy condition. A single health warden
recently ventured to visit a house where smallpox existed in an upper room; he sent for the
attendant, and when she appeared, ordering
her not to approach him, he gave the following
as the best means of prevention: "Burn camphor on the stove, and hang bags of camphor
about the necks of the children."

To what depth of humiliation must that community have descended, which tolerates as its
sanitary officers men who are not only utterly
disqualified by education, business, and moral

character, but who have not even the poor
qualification of courage to perform their duties.
But perhaps the most decisive proof of the utter
and hopeless inefficiency of our multiform
health arrangements is found in the fact that all
the evils from which we now suffer have grown
up under their care. A late City Inspector thus
emphatically gave expression to the popular
feeling in regard to existing organizations:

"With such a system, can there be a wonder
that the sanitary condition of the city is not improved? * * * Nor must the consideration be
kept from view, that the members of the common council, the board of health, and commissioners of health are all, from the manner of
their appointment, subject to partisan influence. To expect a perfect sanitary system,
under such a condition of things, is to expect
an impossibility."

THE medical officer of health for the City of
London, a gentleman of large experience,
thus defines a health organization capable of
answering the demands of a large and growing
town: "The object of this organization lies in
a word: inspection, inspection of
Sanitary the most constant, most searching,
Inspection most intelligent, and most trust-
worthy kind, is that in which the
provisional management of our sanitary affairs
must essentially consist." The results of this

work of voluntary sanitary inspection which I have before me prove on every page the truth of the above statement. No health organization without daily inspection would have any efficiency.

Of the value of such thorough inspection in the suppression of epidemics, and in the prevention of disease, there are abundant examples. The people of a populous town of England, becoming alarmed at the approach of cholera in 1849, organized a corps of inspectors, whose duty it was to visit from house to house, and inquire for cases of premonitory diarrhoea, and when found to apply the remedy at once. The result was that cholera did not visit that town. The same systematic house-to-house visitation was adopted in some poor districts of London in 1854, and there was an almost complete exemption of those parts of the city, while some quarters of the wealthy, which were not under such surveillance, suffered severely.

BUT it is essential that this inspection should be by thoroughly qualified medical men, and it must consist in a house-to-house visitation. Disease must be sought for, found, its incipient history completely made out, the causes upon which it depends reported, and its remedy suggested. Every case of death should be visited, and all the circumstances attending the development

Inspection Must Be Thorough

of the disease, if it belong to the preventable class, should be rigidly investigated and reported, in order that the central bureau may apply the proper remedy.

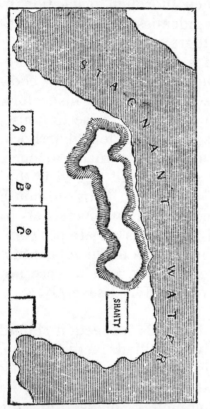

FEVER-BREEDING STAGNANT WATER, EIGHTH AVENUE, BETWEEN 75TH AND 76TH STREETS, 1865

Striking examples of the value of medical sanitary inspection are furnished by this voluntary organization. One inspector found diarrhoeal affections v e r y prevalent in a settlement in an uptown ward, and for a long time was baffled in his efforts to discover the cause. He was finally led to examine the water of a neighboring well, which the people used. This water appeared to be of an excellent quality, but on examination b y Prof. Draper, it was found to contain a large amount of organic matter, derived either from a sewer

or privy. Prof. Draper pronounced it liquid
poison. The mystery was at once solved, and
the proper remedy suggested.

In another instance a very contagious disease
was found in a tenant-house, and after a long
course of inquiry it was at length discovered
that a washer-woman, living in the basement,
had taken in sailors' clothing. The sailors
were found, the ship visited from which they
came, and there the disease was found. None
but medical men can prosecute such investigations with success, or suggest the proper remedy.
If such a corps of sanitary inspectors were
daily patrolling their districts, visiting from
house to house, searching out sanitary evils, ad-
vising and aiding the people in the adoption of
preventive measures, no epidemics of smallpox,
typhus, scarlet fever, or cholera would ever gain
more than a transient foothold. The sanitary
inspector would truly become an officer of
health and would be everywhere welcome.

THE remedy for our evils must be apparent;
and this remedy is suggested in such terse
unqualified language by the City Inspector
above quoted, that I call the attention of the
committee especially to this remark,
The   as a proper guide in your delibera-
Remedy   tions. In the City Inspector's report
for 1861 we find the following:
"The stay of pestilence, to be effectual,

must be prompt, and equally prompt must be the interposition of barriers against the introduction of disease, which may be kept back, but, once introduced, can with difficulty be checked or extirpated. For these reasons, there should be a power existing in other hands that may be ready to be used at the moment the exigency may arise." * * * "The remedy, apparent to every one, must consist in the adoption of laws transferring the power of sanitary regulations to some other authority of a different order of instruction in sanitary science." * * * "The first groundwork of reform, in the opinion of the undersigned, is to bestow upon some other body, differently constituted, all power over the sanitary affairs of the city; and, until this is done, all other proposals of reform will be deprived of their essentially beneficial features. To escape present complications is the first great point to be gained; and this point secured, simplicity, promptness, and efficiency may be substituted for inefficiency, complication, and delay."

Accepting this as the first step in reform, the practical question arises: How shall that body be constituted to which is to be confided the sanitary interests of New York?

IF the experience of other large cities is of any value, or, indeed, if we rely simply on common sense, the following are indispensable prerogatives in any well-organized health board:

1. It should be independent *An Efficient* of all political influence and *Health Board* above all partisan control.

2. It should combine executive ability with a profound knowledge of disease and the proper measures of prevention. To this end the board should be composed in part of men especially accustomed to the dispatch of business, and in part of medical men of great skill and experience.

3. It should have a corps of skilled medical officers as inspectors, which should be the eyes, the ears, in a word, the senses of the board, in every part of the city, searching out disease, investigating the causes which give rise to it, the conditions under which it exists, the means of its propogation, and the most effectual mode of its suppression.

4. It should have a close alliance with the police, which must be its arm of power in the prompt and efficient execution of its orders.

V

Victory

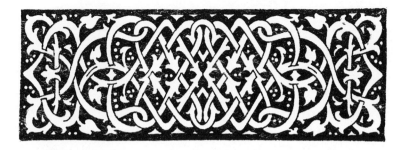

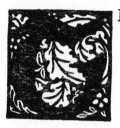HE effect of this startling exhibition of the horrible sanitary condition of New York, both upon the joint committees and the large audience, was evidently very profound. And this effect was heightened by the early denials by the then City Inspector and his followers of the truth of the description of the condition of special localities,

Effect of the Hearing and the immediate exhibitions by the speaker of the sworn statements of the Physician-Inspectors of the Citizens' Association, with photographic illustrations. Pressed by members of the committee to state when he last had these places inspected, he admitted that they had never been inspected by his Department.

Intense interest was manifested in the custom of wholesale dealers in clothing of having their goods manufactured in tenement houses; in the fact that Inspectors had often found such clothing thrown over the beds or cradles of children suffering from contagious diseases, as scarlet

fever, measles, smallpox; and in the evidence
that these diseases were distributed widely over
the country by this infected clothing. Several
of the committee seemed much disturbed, as did
the audience, during a recital of cases, and when
the hearing closed, one of the committee said
to me, in an excited manner, "Why, I bought
underwear at one of those stores a few days
ago, and I believe I have got smallpox, for I
begin to itch all over!"

Indeed, the effect of the discussion before the
joint committees was so favorable, that several
members declared that the bill would immediately pass both Houses without opposition.
But the City Inspector secured delay by request-
ing another hearing, in order to investigate the
facts presented in my quotations from the report of our inspection. This delay gave him
the desired opportunity to defeat the bill, by
means at his command and by methods familiar to that class of politicians.

But the public, and especially the medical profession, both of the city and the State, had become so interested in the measure that at the
next election it became a prominent issue and
led to the defeat of seventeen candidates for the
Legislature of 1866 who had voted in opposition.

IT is said that epidemics are the best promoters
of sanitary reform, and very opportunely
cholera made its dread appearance in Europe

late in 1865, and from its rate of progress it
seemed likely to visit our shores early next
year. These favoring conditions led
Triumph to the passage of the "Metropolitan
at Last Health Law" among the first measures of the Legislature in 1866.

The struggle and final triumph of the people
of New York, in their efforts to secure adequate
health protection, were national in their influence. And this influence was emphasized
by the first acts of the Metropolitan Board.
Scarcely had it organized when cholera made
its appearance in New York. There was the
usual alarm among the people, and large numbers left the city. But the new health laws and
ordinances, administered by an intelligent,
scientific authority, demonstrated the *raison
d'être* of their existence.

The first case of cholera was promptly
isolated, the house and its surroundings
cleansed and disinfected, and rigid supervision
established. The second case, which appeared
in another part of the city, was treated in a
similar manner and with the same results. A
third, fourth, fifth, and finally many cases appeared in different parts of the city during the
season, apparently brought from localities in
the vicinity where the epidemic prevailed with
its usual severity; but in New York no two cases
occurred in the same place, so effectually was
each case treated.

Within one month public confidence in the power of the board to control the spread of the disease was firmly established; people who had fled returned to their homes; business in commercial districts, which was at first suspended, was resumed; and the health department became the most popular branch of the city government, a position which it has maintained uninterruptedly for nearly half a century.

THIS popular triumph of sanitation is largely due to the perfection of the original Metropolitan Law, which has been declared, officially and judicially, to be the most complete piece of health legislation ever placed on the statute books. From that

The Reform National in Its Results

fountain of legal lore the whole country has been supplied with both the principles and the details of sanitary legislation.

The agitation in New York rapidly extended over the entire country, and other cities secured the necessary authority, the Metropolitan Law being the basis of such health legislation. Within a decade nearly every municipality in the land had its health laws and sanitary ordinances and a competent authority to enforce them.

The enormous influence which this reform has had upon the health and domestic life of the people can never be estimated. A reference to the former and present sickness and death-rates of New York enables us to approximate the vast saving of life and consequent prevention of sickness and human misery that has resulted from health laws founded on the Metropolitan Law and intelligently but rightly enforced. Before the passage of that law the annual death-rate of the city fluctuated between 28 and 40 per 1,000 population; since that law went into effect it has steadily fallen until it has reached the low figure of fifteen to the thousand, or a saving of more than twenty thousand lives annually when the population of New York was only about one million, and of nearly 10,000 lives of the present population. If we extend this estimate to the whole country, of ninety-five million people, we may gain a faint conception of the inestimable benefits which the application of sanitary knowledge to the daily life of a people can accomplish.

VI

THE LEGAL WORK OF DORMAN BRIDGEMAN EATON

The following chapter consists of the address delivered by Dr. Stephen Smith on the occasion of the memorial service of Hon. Dorman B. Eaton, January 21, 1899. We have inserted it immediately following his historic review of the events which led up to the great public health reform of 1865-1866, not only because it is a fitting tribute to the memory of one to whom the citizens of New York are indebted for many improvements in the administration of the municipal government, but because it brings together in one compact perspective the legal and sanitary requirements of modern preventive medicine. — F. A.

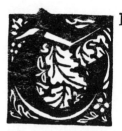HE progress of the race is largely affected in each generation by a few pioneers who, with toil and sacrifice, prepare the way for the advance. Of these pioneers some blaze the future course in the unexplored and trackless forest; others remove the obstructions which impede the builders; while a few expert

Unrecognized Pioneers engineers bridge the rivers, tunnel the mountains and lay broad and deep the foundations of the great highway along which humanity passes to a higher civilization. Unfortunately these pioneers are not always known to public fame, and far too often, though benefactors of their race, pass away without a proper recognition of their services.

This apparent neglect is not due to a lack of appreciation of their work by the people, but rather to the fact that their labors are performed in obscurity, and hence are unknown. Far in the wilderness, or deep in the tunnel, or in the mire of the caisson, they toil all unseen

by their generation, sacrificing health and often
life while seaching for the true pathway or lay-
ing its foundations. When the bridges are
builded, the tunnels completed, and the broad
highway is thrown open for travel and traffic,
few or none of the passing throng give a moment's thought to the labors and sacrifices of
the builders, or the tribute of a sigh to the memory of those who perished at their work.

Impressed with a sense of public obligation
and of a duty to the memory of a citizen with
whose labors and sacrifices in the interests of
this city I had great opportunities to become familiar, it has been a grateful task to place on
record some of the incidents in the life of Hon.
Dorman B. Eaton as they came under my personal observation.   He was by nature, education, and association a reformer of the civil administration.   Born and bred in the rural communities of Vermont, educated at Harvard, a
partner of the famous Judge Kent, of this city,
and an associate of men of the type of William
Curtis Noyes, Charles O'Conor, and others of
equal reputation, Mr. Eaton was admirably
equipped for the great work to which he devoted so much of his life and energies.

NOR was he a reformer whose methods were
simply destructive of what he regarded as
wrong or evil in the municipal government;
on the contrary, his mind was eminently con-

structive, and consequently he sought to remedy defects by substituting the new *A Constructive Reformer* and best for the old and worst with as little friction and disturbance as possible. Thus he quietly and without observation, as a master builder, laid foundations and reared the massive superstructures of four of the best-organized and most efficient departments of our city government — viz., the Department of Health, the Fire Department, the Department of Docks, the Police Judiciary.

M Y personal acquaintance with Mr. Eaton began in the year 1864, when we became associated in an effort to secure reforms in the sanitary government of the City of New York. Although prior to this date there had been periods of agitation in favor of a more *Character of Previous Agitation* efficient health organization, especially when epidemics, like cholera, visited the city and the utter worthlessness of our health officials became apparent, yet there had been no such organized effort as that of 1864. Previous agitation had, however, been very useful in preparing the way for the final struggle, by creating a popular interest in these reforms and in rendering the public mind both sympathetic and receptive.

I N 1855 the Academy of Medicine applied to the Legislature for relief from the evils of an insufficient health organization, and as a result a committee of that body investigated the sanitary condition of the city. It appeared that there were four separate de-

Incompetent Health Officers partments devoted to the conservation of the public health. First, was the Board of Health, composed of the Aldermen and Mayor. When this body was organized as a Board of Health it had supreme power, both in the abatement of nuisances and the expenditure of money. So much and so justly was this board feared, that Fernando Wood, while Mayor, refused to call it into existence during an epidemic of cholera, declaring that the Board of Health was more to be feared than the pestilence.

Second, was the Commissioners of Health, composed of the Mayor and the Recorder, the City Inspector, the Health Commissioner, the Resident Physician, and the Port Health Officer. This body had no adequate power and was perfectly useless both for good and evil.

Third, was the Resident Physician, whose duties were limited to visiting the sick poor.

Fourth, was the City Inspector, a most formidable official politically, for he had the right to expend annually $1,000,000 without "let or hindrance." His jurisdiction extended to the cleaning of the street, gathering vital statistics, and preserving the public health by the appointment of health wardens for each ward.

The investigation showed that this department, the only one which actually exercised public health functions, was permeated with corruption, ignorance, and venality. The City Inspector was the lowest type of ward politician, the vital statistics were crude and unreliable, there was no pretense of cleaning the streets, and the health wardens were for the most part keepers of saloons. It was shown in the evidence that no health warden ever dared to visit a house where there was a case of contagious disease. One, who was asked the best method of preventing smallpox, replied: "Burn sulphur in the room." Another, asked to define the term "hygiene," said: "It is a mist rising from wet grounds."

THE report of this committee created a profound sensation and gave the first impetus to a reform movement. A number of prominent physicians and influential citizens became deeply interested in the subject and determined to secure proper legislation. Health bills

Reform Movement Born

were annually prepared and sent to the Legislature only to be rejected under the direction of the City Inspector, whose $1,000,000 was expended freely in the lobby at Albany. But the agitation increased in force with successive defeats, a large and still larger number of people were added to the ranks of the reformers of the Citizens' Association in 1864, with Peter Cooper as President and upwards of a hundred of the leading citizens as members.

The moving spirit in organizing and managing this powerful body was Mr. Nathaniel Sands, an ardent and enthusiastic sanitarian. Two departments were created in the Association, through which the principal work was to be done; viz., a Council of Law and a Council of Hygiene. Mr. Eaton was an active member of the former, and I was for a considerable time Secretary of the latter. Thus we were brought into frequent consultation over a public health law, which the Association had determined to have prepared for the next Legislature.

It was decided that the Council of Hygiene should make a first draft of the bill in which should be incorporated the necessary sanitary provisions. This draft was then to be submitted to the Legal Council for completion in legislative form. As secretary of the Council of Hygiene I had to prepare the first draft of the bill, which was done along the lines of former bills and seemed to the members to be a very perfect piece of work. When, however, the bill came from the Legal Council, scarcely a shred of the original draft was recognizable.

THOUGH the Legal Council was composed of the leading lawyers of the city at that time, the revision and completion of the health law was committed to Mr. Eaton, a junior member. This selection proved to be of immense importance to the immediate sanitary interests of this city, and secondarily to the creation and administration of the health laws of the United States. The field of sanitary legislation was entirely uncultivated in this country at that time, and the principles on which health laws should be based were unrecognized, except by the more advanced students.

The Right Man

Mr. Eaton fortunately proved to be one of the few citizens who had kept pace with the progress of sanitary reforms in England, and entered fully into the spirit of the great movement that for a quarter of a century had agitated the people of that country. Alarmed by the high death-rate annually reported by the Registrar-General, and informed that the larger part was due to preventable diseases, the public demanded adequate remedial measures of the government. The contest was long and most exciting, the issues often being carried into the arena of politics. The Prime Minister once declared that there was such a craze about sanitation that the rallying cry of an election campaign might well be *"Sanitas sanitatum, et omnia sanitas."*

The triumph of the reformers was finally complete, and England adopted a code of health laws that are models of excellence, and which, in their enforcement, have made its cities and towns the healthiest in the world.

When our health bill came from the hands of Mr. Eaton it was evident in every line that he had made an exhaustive study of the English health code and had become thoroughly imbued with its spirit. The language was not altogether familiar, and in the involved sentences there were intimations of extraordinary powers quite unknown to our jurisprudence. When he brought the completed bill before the Legal and Medical councils for adoption it was subjected to a most searching criticism. While most of its sections were clear and readily understood, there were portions which were so obscure, owing to the methods of expression employed, that the legal members were in doubt as to the proper construction to be put upon them, while the medical members were altogether at a loss as to their meaning.

MR. EATON explained the theory of modern health legislation as illustrated by the English laws, and contended that a thoroughly organized and efficient board of health must have extraordinary powers, and must not be subordinated to any other branch of the civil service, not even to the courts. What it declared to be a nuisance — dangerous to life and detrimental to health — no one should call in question. When it ordered a nuisance to be abated within a given fixed time no mandate should avail to stay its action or the enforcement of its decree.

A Board With Extraordinary Powers

A board of health, in his opinion, should make its own laws, execute its own laws, and sit in judgment on its own acts. It must be an *imperium in imperio.* England, the foremost country in the world in the cultivation of sanitary science and in the application of its principles to practice, had by its legislation for a quarter of a century established a precedent which it was right and safe for us to follow.

He predicted that if this bill became a law its operations would be so beneficial that it would not only become very popular in this city, but that it would be the basis of future health legislation in this country. He believed, however, that no legislature would pass a bill containing such powers if these powers were made a prominent feature of the bill. For that reason he had adopted that involved expression peculiar to English law which required a judicial interpretation to determine the precise meaning. The bill was approved in the form presented by Mr. Eaton, and preparation was made to secure its passage.

A S the City Inspector with his health wardens
always appeared at Albany when a health
bill was before the Legislature, denying
vociferously the alleged unsanitary condition of
the city, Mr. Eaton advised that the Association
make a careful inspection of the
The Fight for city with its own inspectors.
the Bill   This inspection was organized
by the Council of Hygiene and
prosecuted during the summer of 1864 by young
physicians, and was the most exhaustive study
of the sanitary condition ever made of a city,
even by officials. The results were published in
a large volume which has been pronounced by
authorities at home and abroad as equal to the
best official reports of European cities.

The bill was early introduced into the Legislature of 1865. In due time it came before a joint
committee of both houses, with Senator Andrew
D. White in the chair. The City Inspector, with
his health wardens, was present, and a large at-
tendance of members with several prominent
citizens of New York. At Mr. Eaton's request
I described the deplorable sanitary condition of
the city as revealed by our inspections and explained the medical features of the bill. He
followed with a brilliant and exhaustive speech
on the nature of sanitary legislation and the
value to cities of adequate health laws administered by well-organized boards of health.

At the conclusion of the hearing the members

of the committee assured us that if the two
houses were in session they would pass the bill
at once.   But we were doomed to disappoint-
ment.   The City Inspector secured delays, and
meantime employed through his agents the
means at his command to defeat the bill.   The
agitation, however, was continued during the
year, chiefly through the *New York Times,* then
under the management of Mr. Raymond, an
ardent reformer.

MR. EATON advised the Medical Council to
interest the physicians of the country, and
especially urge them not to nominate men
who had voted against the bill in the last Legislature.   This plan was carried out, and seventeen former members failed
A Law Enacted   of renomination to the As-
and Sustained   sembly.   The result of this
scheme succeeded admirably,
for the new Legislature was to some extent
pledged to support the bill when they came to
the capitol.   The bill promptly passed both
houses early in the session of 1866, and in
March the Metropolitan Board of Health was
organized.   Mr. Eaton accepted the position of
counsellor to the board, which position he retained several years.

As he had anticipated, a suit against the Board
was early commenced to test the constitu-
tionality of the law.   He was very apprehensive

of the results, and made the most thorough preparation to argue the case. He was successful in the lower courts, and finally won in the Court of Appeals by a majority of one. He always regarded his success in the management of this case as one of the most important events of his life, for on the decision of the highest court depended the fate of health legislation in this country.

N O one unfamiliar with the sanitary condition of this city prior to 1864 can form any adequate conception of the enormous benefits conferred, not only upon this metropolis, but upon the entire country, by the labors of Mr. Eaton and his associates in securing to it the Metropolitan Health Law. During the former period New York was a prey to every form of pestilence known to man. Smallpox, the most preventable of contagious diseases, was epidemic in this city every five years, and created a large death-rate among the children. Scarlet fever and diphtheria spread through the city without the slightest effort on the part of the officials to control them. Cholera visited us once in ten years without any adequate measures of prevention. The mortality was greater than of any other city of a civilized country, it being estimated that 7,000 died yearly from preventable diseases.

The Regeneration of New York

The tenement-house population lived under the most unhealthy and degrading conditions, a prey to greedy landlords, and without any possible relief or redress. In one notorious building, which covered an ordinary city lot, were fifty families, with a total population of five hundred persons.

Here every form of domestic pestilence could be found at all seasons of the year. Still more deplorable was the condition of the tenants of cellars. Of these so-called "Troglodytes" there were 5,000 living in rooms the ceilings of which were below the level of the surface of the street.

To the present generation it may appear incredible that there was neither law, ordinance, nor department of the city government capable of giving the slightest relief. This was illustrated in an attempt to break up a fever nest in 1860. The landlord refused to make the slightest repairs, or cleansing, in a tenement house from which upwards of one hundred cases of fever have been removed to the hospital.

The attorney to the Police Department was unable to find any law or ordinance by which he could be compelled to cleanse, repair, or vacate the house. It was only by confronting him in court, to which he had been brought on a fictitious charge, with a reporter, that he was induced to take any steps to improve the tenement.

NOW everything relating to the public health is so changed that it is almost impossible to realize the condition of the city in 1866. The change began with the very organization of the Metropolitan Board. Within a few days of that event, cholera, which had dev-

Epidemics astated portions of Europe, made *Checked* its appearance in this city; but it met with a far different reception than that of former visitations. The first case was quarantined within an hour of its occurrence; the clothing of the patient was destroyed, the room disinfected, and a sanitary guard placed over the house. No other case appeared in that quarter of the city. There were several similar outbreaks in different parts of the town, but each was treated with the same vigilance and energy, and the contagion never secured a foothold in the city or the metropolitan district.

Though cholera has since appeared in Europe at its usual intervals, and has several times been at our doors, it has not been able to invade the city for a period of thirty-four years. Smallpox, which once decimated the child population every five years, has not been epidemic in a whole generation. Diphtheria and the whole brood of domestic pestilences are diminishing in frequency and fatality. Even consumption, so common and fatal among the poor, is rapidly disappearing in consequence of the improved condition of the tenement houses.

And what a vast change has been made in the homes of the poor! No human habitation is underground; the ancient rookery, with its five hundred inhabitants, is a past number; the dark, foul courts are disappearing, and in their places have arisen the modern tenements, with their light, airy, and cheerful apartments, and all the conditions necessary to family health and domestic happiness. The laws and ordinances all conspire to compel the landlords to remedy every defect on complaint of the tenant; the penalty being that the latter need not pay rent until the home is made habitable in a sanitary sense. The vital statistics show that human life is lengthening in this city, and that the entire metropolis is more healthy as a place of residence than the sorrounding country towns.

BUT the beneficent results of the labors of Mr. Eaton and his associates in the field of sanitary legislation are not confined to New York. As he predicted, the Metropolitan Health Law became the basis of sanitary legislation throughout the country. At the time of its enactment the municipalities of the United States were as destitute of health laws and regulations as the City of New York. Today there is not a city, or even village, that has not its laws and ordinances relating to the preservation and promotion of the public health

Sanitation in Other Cities

based on the original law drawn by Mr. Eaton.
And the same remark is true of the organized
health administration of the States of the Union,
for on analysis it will be found that their sanitary legislation is in harmony with the provisions of that law. Mr. Eaton's work was broad
and fundamental.

AT that period the old Volunteer Fire Depart-
   was quite as discreditable to the city as was
its health organization. Intrenched in the
political organizations of the city, it wielded a
power second only to that of the great political
parties themselves. It
Reorganization of the required the strength
Fire Department and courage of a Her-
cules to purify this de-
partment by removing the existing elements, re-
constructing the entire organization, substituting a paid for a volunteer membership, and requiring a high grade of qualification of its
officers.

   But, aided by the Citizens' Association, Mr.
Eaton undertook this reform, and after a
fierce and prolonged struggle carried it to a
successful conclusion. The law creating the
fire department, like that creating the health department, is a model of intelligent discrimination of all the conditions essential to the efficiency of the service and its permanent freedom from the vices inherent in the old system.

SCARCELY had these reforms been perfected when Mr. Eaton's attention was turned by the Citizens' Association to the necessity of having a department in the city government devoted exclusively to the care and management of the p u b l i c d o c k s, *Creation of a Dock* wharves, and other water-*Department* front interests of the city. This movement resulted in the passage of the law drawn by Mr. Eaton creating the Department of Docks. Though this Department was to occupy an entirely new field in the Municipal Administration, the law shows in every section the same mastery of all the details peculiar to Mr. Eaton's legislative work.

FINALLY, Mr. Eaton undertook, single-handed, to reform the police judiciary. He prepared a bill creating the civil magistrates to take the place of the police justices and reforming in many particulars the methods of procedure. This law is regarded *Reform of the* as a great improvement upon *Police Judiciary* the previous police judiciary, but the bill became a law only after a protracted struggle with the old police justices, a struggle which Mr. Eaton maintained alone, relying upon the merits of the measure which he advocated. The consensus of opinion of legal authorities is that the new law effected

radical reforms of great importance in these in-
ferior courts of criminal jurisprudence in New
York City.

I F we may estimate Mr. Eaton's mental traits
by the laws which he drafted in the interests
of municipal reform, we can readily conclude
that he had a remarkable genius for constructive
legislation. Though he was compelled to weave
into the very woof of those
Mental Traits of laws, extraordinary powers,
Dorman B. Eaton which he acknowledged
were of vital importance to
their efficiency, and yet would be a menace to
the public, if the laws were administered by
unscrupulous persons, he succeeded in so
guarding those powers that these laws have
been in operation upwards of a quarter of a century; and, while those who have from time to
time been called to administer them have not
always had the best reputation for intelligence
and civic virtue, yet there has at no time been
any complaint of injustice in their execution,
nor has there been any serious lapse in their
vigorous enforcement. To-day, as a generation
ago, they are accomplishing the full measure of
usefulness for which they were designed by
their author.

Standing now at the close of a life so largely
devoted to the service of his fellow-men and
consecrated to the amelioration of human suf-

fering, and where we may, in some slight degree, estimate the vast and ever-increasing
fruition of its labors, how sublime it appears!
Monuments and memorials can but faintly sym-
bolize its greatness and perpetuate its enduring
force. Mr. Eaton's own thought of true fame
once was expressed to me thus: "I ask only to
be remembered as one who in his sphere of life's
duties endeavored to improve the conditions of
human life around him."

VII
THE OCCULT POWER OF FILTH

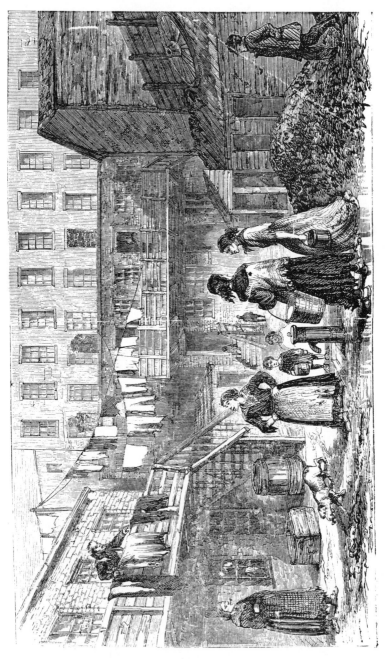

THE DRY HYDRANT. BAXTER STREET.

N the retrospect from the vantage ground of half a century of sanitary progress we recognize that during the third quarter of the last century the people of England were waging a successful war on domestic uncleanliness as a contributory, if not the sole cause of epidemic diseases. The health officer of England insisted that domestic filth was the actual cause of many of the low forms of disease, and named them accordingly, "filth diseases." This official act of the highest health authority of that country led to the practice of cleanliness in the home and its surroundings. Filth in every form was removed as the necessary remedial measure against these diseases, with the result that not only were foreign pestilences prevented, but the whole brood of domestic diseases was greatly reduced in number, and the severity of cases that did occur was greatly diminished in virulence.

Filth Diseases

But during the fourth quarter of the last cen-

tury the question arose among scientists, "Why
is filth — that is, decomposing matter — the
prolific cause of disease?" The answer came
from the famous Pasteur of Paris, and Lister
of Edinburgh. "Filth is dangerous, because it
is filled with germ life. The mere removal of
filth from one locality to another does not
render it harmless, except to those who are no
longer in personal contact with it." So-called
filth was indeed harmless if the germs it contained were killed.

THE whole scheme of sanitation was at once
changed: agents that would kill germs were
eagerly sought by many scientists, and
germicides were found in abundance. Crema-
tion was most effectful,
and was available in the
destruction of masses of
filth; but there was a
phase of the question that required other methods.

*The Scheme of
Sanitation Changed*

Lister announced that these disease-producing germs entered wounds and prevented heal-
ing, and that a germicide was required which
would kill the germ in the wound and would
not injure the living, healthy tissue. Further
investigations showed that these dangerous
germs were not confined to dust heaps, but
existed in the unclean recesses of the human
body.

Sternberg startled the world with the announcement that an unclean human mouth contained germs of the most poisonous character.

An eminent German surgeon declared that germs of a dangerous character existed in the folds of the skin of the palms of the hand which no amount of washing with soap and water could remove, and could be destroyed only by some agent directly applied.

Sanitation of the body as well as of the dust heap now became the paramount question and especially did this apply to the practice of surgery.

HOW infection affects the body was the supreme mystery that the scientists of the past strove in vain to penetrate. By no devices of their laboratories could they detect the agents that caused the epidemic. There was only one satisfactory explanation of the origin and spread of *The Mystery of Infection* the devastating plagues, which seemed to fall from the heavens on the people, and that was that epidemics were "a visitation of God" on account of the sins of the people. Of course, the only preventive and curative measure available and effectual was "repentance, prayer, and humiliation."

It is a cause of devout thankfulness that while these things were hidden from the "wise and

prudent" of former times, they have in these
latter days been revealed unto "babes." No
event in human history would have more greatly
taxed the credulity of the most learned and experienced physician of half a century ago than
the prophecy that in the early years of the twentieth century school children would be taught
by simple and easily understood object lessons
how to prevent and how to cure consumption,
the Asiatic cholera, yellow fever, and other epidemics that have devastated cities, destroyed
armies, and swept from the earth whole tribes
of primitive people.

But that prophecy has been literally fulfilled.
During the last summer there has been a travel-
ing object lesson that visited the different sections of the State of New York and taught the
people, especially the children, all the essential
facts as to the nature of the infection of tuberculosis, its effects on the body, and the methods
of prevention and cure.

A S infective diseases cause the vast majority
of cases of severe and crippling affections
and of deaths in every community, the
value of a knowledge of the nature of infection
and how it affects the body, by the people of all
ranks, ages, and conditions, cannot be estimated
in its influence on the future of the human race.
Already we learn that within the period referred
to the sickness and death-rates of communities

where the people have been most thoroughly in-
                        structed as to the nature of in-
How Infection fective diseases, and how they
    Works   affect the body, have greatly
                        diminished, and the average
human life has been markedly lengthened.
Indeed, it now seems possible to restore the patriarchal age when a man
may live to be "an hundred and twenty
years old . . . his eye . . . not dim, nor his
natural force abated."

To understand how infection affects the body
involves an inquiry as to the nature of infection,
its mode of entrance into the body, and its
operation on its organs and tissues. The terms
"infection" and "contagion" are often used as
synonymous; but a strict definition according
to the medical significance of each limits the
former to "the transmission of disease by actual
contact of the diseased part with a healthy ab-
sorbent or abraded surface," and the latter to
"transmission through the atmosphere by floating germs." But in the final analysis the cause
of disease in both infection and contagion is so
similar in its action that the medical profession
has adopted the term "communicable disease"
in all cases where the disease is communicated
from one person to another by means of a
germ, whatever may be its method of attack on
the body. The common characteristic of "communicable diseases" is their germ origin.

W HAT is this communicable germ or agent?
A bacterium — a little stick, staff — so
called from the rodlike shape it assumes
in the process of growth. The individual bacterium (plural, bacteria) is an organism representing a low form of vegetable
What the life; resembles mold; in size the
Germ Is smallest living thing that can be
seen with the microscope; in
masses forming the films floating on foul fluids
or covering decomposing animal or vegetable
matter. It consists of a single cell, and its mode
of increase when placed under proper conditions of growth is by division of the cell body;
the two cells formed out of the first being divided into four before complete separation has
taken place; the four dividing into eight, the
eight into sixteen, the sixteen into thirty-two,
and so on indefinitely.

Now, as it requires only thirty minutes for
one cell to divide, it has been estimated that a
single bacterium will in twenty-four hours increase to the number of over sixteen million
five hundred thousand, and in forty-eight hours
to two hundred and eighty-one million five hundred thousand. At this rate of increase, in three
days there would be a mass of bacteria weigh-
ing about sixteen million pounds. As the multiplication of bacteria depends upon conditions
that soon interfere with or interrupt their
growth, as the want of food, their own secre-

tions, and certain natural forces operating against them, these stupendous figures are useful only as an illustration of the enormous fertility of these organisms, and their destructive energy when they attack a susceptible living body.

WHAT is the function of bacteria in the economy of nature? It would be surprising if such a menace to human life as some species of bacteria have proved themselves to be had no other place among the forces of nature than to prevent the *The Function of* too rapid increase of the *Bacteria* human race on this earth, as our forefathers believed. It is gratifying, and quite satisfying to a revengeful spirit, to learn from the modern laboratory that the special and only function of the bacterium is to perform the duties of a universal scavenger. It is always seeking to decompose animal and vegetable matter. It lives on filth, riots in it, and dies when deprived of it. It enters the human body only in search of filth, and if it finds none it does the person no harm, and dies either from the want of food or by starvation, or escapes from the body, or secretes itself where it may safely await the creation of decomposing matter, when it will begin its lifework.

Thus, there may be and doubtless is at all

times a great variety of bacteria of a virulent type, quiescent in our bodies only for the time that they find no decaying matter adapted to their special tastes or wants.

It is a most interesting fact, therefore, that this most deadly foe of man becomes dangerous only when the latter is harboring in his body waste or decomposing matters that are slowly poisoning him. It is in the process of digesting this material that the bacterium excretes poisons — toxins — of the most virulent nature, which are absorbed into the blood of the human victim, creating the condition popularly known as blood poisoning.

Bacteria perform a most important function in the economy of nature, viz., the conversion of decaying and dead matter into food for plants. Biologists assert that without bacteria plant life on the earth would be scanty or entirely wanting; they are the natural intermediaries between plants and animal in point of food production. They are therefore called scavengers, because they live on decomposing matter; but in the very act of digesting such waste they convert it into products essential to plant life (carbon dioxide and ammonia) and by their excretions restore to vegetation its chief supply of food.

It appears on the same authorities that bacteria not only assist materially in maintaining vegetable and animal life on this planet, but

"in the arts and industries they are as essential
to modern economic life as are the ingenious
mechanical inventions of men.   Many secret
processes now in use in the arts and manufac-
tures are but devices to harness these natural
forces.   Thus in the manufacture of linen,
hemp, and sponges, in the butter, cheese, and
vinegar industries, in tobacco-curing, etc., bacteria play an important rôle."

IT naturally occurs that to meet the various
conditions under which decomposing matter
exists in nature there is a great variety of
species of bacteria, each species being adapted
to a special field of operations.   These species
                     are distinguished from one
Bacteria for   another by the shapes they
Every Condition   assume during their growth,
                     some being rod shaped (the
bacillus), others spherical (the coccus), and
others spiral (the spirillum).   Under one of
these divisions the various species are classified.

In these latter days of popular knowledge of
scientific progress, but without precise information of details, bacteria are associated in the
public mind with disease, especially of the epidemic form.   While this prejudice is useful
in stimulating the people to adopt and enforce
preventive measures against conditions that
tend to promote bacterial life in their homes
and in their own persons, yet it should be un-

derstood that comparatively few of the great
number and variety of bacteria are pathogenic,
or disease producing, in man.

So throughout the animal kingdom we find
that few are susceptible to a common disease;
or, in other words, that the same species of bacteria attack in equal force several varieties of
animals.

The explanation of this peculiarity is found
in the variations of the quality or intimate nature of the tissues and organs of different species of animals. The same may be said of our
own bodies — the several organs vary greatly
in their susceptibility to the attacks of the different kinds of bacteria; hence the latter are
classified as specific and nonspecific, according
as they cause specific or nonspecific disease.

The distribution of bacteria is limited only by
the existence of plants and animals; that is, the
existence of decomposing vegetable and animal
matter. Though they are more abundant in the
earth where such matter is found most abundantly, yet they abound in the air, the water, on
plants, animals, and insects, on our own bodies,
and in every cavity leading to the exterior. As
bacteria are always searching for food, the number present is a sure indication of the degree of
cleanliness of the thing, individual, or locality
where they are found.

The movements of bacteria from one point
to another are through the medium of some

other mode of conveyance than their own bodies afford. Thus they are borne by the water, by vegetation, by animals of every kind, especially insects, by the air on particles of dust. The typhoid bacillus, borne in water and milk, has caused innumerable epidemics of that dreaded disease.

THE tubercle bacillus is borne on the air through the medium of particles of dust, and in cities where the victims of tuberculosis scatter these germs profusely in the streets, public conveyances, churches, and places of resort, in the act of *The Deadly* coughing, sneezing, and spit- *Tubercle Bacillus* ting, the dust borne on the winds is a constant and most fertile source of infection of tuberculosis. In a city like New York thousands are annually infected by the dust-borne tubercle bacilli, not only by inhaling them in the street, but even more certainly in the quiet of their homes, where the germ-bearing dust accumulates in clothing, bedding, carpets, rugs, and upholstered furniture, and is daily forced into the air of the living rooms by broom and duster.

Foul as is the air of the unventilated tenements of the poor, it has been demonstrated that the dust which saturates the furniture, carpets, rugs, and hangings of residences of the wealthy contains sixty per cent of street filth.

An authority says, "The most widely distributed pathogenic microörganism (disease-
causing bacterium) in the air is the tubercle
bacillus, the cause of consumption and a large
variety of other ailments, such as hipjoint disease, caries of the spine, etc. Over one hundred
thousand persons die annually from consumption alone in the United States, and it is estimated that there are over two million people
afflicted with the disease in one form or another. All of these sufferers are expectorating
billions of tubercle bacilli daily."

CONSIDERING the second inquiry as to how
infection affects the body, we must constantly bear in mind that a bacterium,
though a scavenger, is a conservator of nature.
Its real function in the orderly processes of
animal and vegetable life is
How Bacteria to utilize waste for the pre-
Affect the Body servation and promotion of
animal and vegetable life on
this planet where the conditions are so favorable to both.

Therefore, wherever we find bacteria in the
active processes of growth, that is, multiplication, we may be assured that they have found
matter that should be rescued from waste and
converted into useful food for plants. It follows
that when we find a bacterium actively growing
in any part of our bodies, it has found some

form of decaying matter that is not only no longer useful to our bodies, but is in fact harmful and should be removed.

It is also important to understand that waste matter is found under a great variety of conditions, and that for its proper conversion into useful food for plants there must be a correspondingly large number of species of bacteria each having its special field of operation. It is due to this variety of bacteria that there are so many infective diseases; for each species of bacteria creates its own individual form of disease.

This statement requires the following explanation, viz., a bacterium in a quiescent state is harmless; everyone has within his body innumerable bacteria, as the tubercle and typhoid bacilli; but they are inert, and hence innocuous. It is only when they find their proper food, decaying matter, that they begin to multiply, and in that act they secret a poison, toxin, which is absorbed, and, entering the circulation, causes in the individual a special class of symptoms peculiar to that toxin, or poison.

These symptoms constitute a disease, the technical name of which is usually fanciful, depending on some feature of the symptoms, but explaining nothing as to its essential nature.

For example, the typhoid bacillus finds its food in certain minute glands of the small bowels. If these glands are in a perfectly healthy state when the bacillus enters the digestive tract, the germ will pass over them and disappear from the body perfectly harmless. But if the bacillus finds its appropriate food — dead or decomposing matter — in the glands, it at once takes up its abode in them and "begins housekeeping;" that is, it begins to multiply according to the method of fission of its cell and rate of multiplication, already described. During this process the multiplying cells excrete a toxin, which, being absorbed, creates a fever, the result of a true blood poisoning. This fever is called typhoid, because its prominent symptom, stupor, resembles that of typhus fever. The name, therefore, signifies nothing as to the nature of the disease.

THE poisoning of the body by the excreted toxin of the multiplying cells, which is simply plant food, occurs because it is removed only in part by the digestive organs, the circulation that conveys it to the other eliminating organs being efficient for that

The Toxin purpose. Could all of this toxin
Secreted be removed as fast as it is excreted, and not enter the circulation, there would be no fever.

The termination of this process must be either the death of the colony from exhaustion of the food supply in the glands, or the exhaustion of the patient by the excess of toxins that ac-

cumulate in the body.. As the activity of the
bacillus depends upon the food supplied, the
severity and length of the fever varies in different individuals. Some are immune, because
the glands that furnish the food of the typhoid
bacillus are in a state of high health; others
have a brief and mild attack, because the food
supply is scant owing to a slight impairment
of the integrity of the glands; but with a considerable number in every epidemic the food is
ample to sustain the creation of an immense
colony of bacilli which destroys the victim by
an overdose of poison.

The final disposition of the typhoid bacilli,
after a course of fever, was believed to be by
their elimination from the body through the
various organs devoted to the discharge of waste
products; but recent investigations have proved
that the typhoid bacillus may remain in the
body for long periods without apparently affecting the health of the person, but when communicated to another, it will cause an attack
of fever of the most virulent type. In one instance an outbreak of typhoid fever was traced
to a woman who had fever upward of fifty
years ago. It was found that the excretions of
her body contained immense quantities of living
typhoid bacilli. She was a cook by trade, and it
was found on tracing her history that wherever
she had worked there had been epidemics of
typhoid.

A still more remarkable feature of the life
history of the typhoid bacillus has recently
been made public. A typhoid epidemic was
traced to a nurse who had attended cases of
typhoid fever, but had never suffered from an
attack of that disease, and yet was discharging
large quantities of the bacilli. These cases can
be explained only on the theory that these
microörganisms find some place, possibly, as
has been suggested, in the gall bladder, where
they find food sufficient to keep them in an
active state of multiplication, but where the conditions prevent the absorption of the toxins
they excrete.

How far these curious incidents in the life
of the typhoid bacilli are common to other
bacilli is not known; but if it is true of other
infectious diseases, the fact will explain the
origin of those obscure and mysterious cases
that occur without any known exposure to the
infection.

IN concluding this inquiry as to the nature of
infection and its effects on the body, the following statement of a biologist as to the bacterium seems justified: "When it enters a living
body, it aims directly at the destruction of the
latter. It multiplies rapidly, tends to scatter its
broods throughout the tissues, and all the while
gives off the most powerful poisons. This agent
is wickedly implacable, neither giving nor ask-

ing quarter. The battle that it wages with the body can terminate only by the destruction of one of the combatants."

Bacteria Aim to Destroy the Body

Viewed in the light of the past history of infectious diseases, this is not an overdrawn picture. If we estimate the deaths from smallpox in ancient times, from cholera in modern times, and from tuberculosis (consumption) throughout all time, the destruction of human life by bacteria cannot be overstated. The bacterium has been a wickedly implacable foe to the human race in the past. Invisible, intangible, everywhere present, it has proved omnipotent in its destructive attacks upon communities.

But our century opens with a far brighter outlook for the race. Elementary forces which, through ignorance of their true functions in the economy and conservation of nature, were permitted in the past to expend their energy in the destruction of life, have been revealed by science to be man's most helpful agents in the promotion of comfort, health, and longevity. Electricity was for ages only a thunderbolt, an object of terror, and an agent of destruction, visiting the human residence only to kill its owner and burn the structure.

To-day the same natural force is man's most obedient and humble servant, quietly visiting his home to furnish him heat and light, annihi-

lating time in the transactions of business, and
transporting him from place to place as on the
lightning's wings.

So the bacterium, once the terror of mankind
as the invisible and apparently unknowable
cause of devastating pestilences, proves to be
the useful purveyor of the by-products of man's
digestion of waste matter which is thereby converted into food for plants. It visits man in the
pursuit of its humble calling to obtain his con-
tribution to the sum total of plant food. It
searches every tissue, every organ, every recess,
however obscure, but so stealthily that its coming and going and its immediate presence are
not known if absolute cleanliness of the body
exists. It is only when dying tissues or organs,
or accumulations of dead matter, are found that
its presence becomes known. Even then it
would prove harmless and its presence would
be unrecognized if its excretions of plant food
(toxins) were not necessarily absorbed and did
not enter the circulation, thus poisoning the
body it is relieving of dead matter.

BRIEFLY, what are man's defenses against
bacteria? Chiefly two, viz., first, killing it
by depriving it of food; and, second, killing
it directly by what are known as germicides.
The first method is effected by cleanliness of
the person. It may be affirmed that cleanliness,
without and within, absolutely protects every

man, woman, and child from the most common disease-producing bacteria.

Man's   It is not sufficient to keep the skin
Defenses   clean by daily baths, while the
                  mouth, nose, throat, and other
internal surfaces and organs are covered or filled with effete matter. We must be every whit clean if we would escape the results of the scavenging processes of bacteria of some variety or species.

That condition can be secured and maintained in an organism that itself is constantly decaying in all of its tissues and organs only by strict compliance with the natural laws governing the operations of the body as an independent organism in which all of its forces tend to promote its health and conservation. Every tissue and every organ has its special means of renewal of its tissue by the removal of dead particles through the outlets and the reception of fresh material through the inlets of the body. Waste and supply are exactly balanced, as in the most precise and delicate machine. If the outlets become clogged, so that all the waste cannot escape at that proper time, dead matter, the food of bacteria, begins to accumulate, and disease must result.

In the same manner, if the food is in excess of the demands, or of a quality not suited to the needs of the tissue or organ, waste begins to accumulate, bacteria swarm in the decomposing

mass, and emit their toxins, which, absorbed
into the circulation, cause a variety of physical
disturbances according to the species of bacteria present, and the particular tissues the
toxins affect, as the nervous system, stomach,
heart, kidneys, etc.

That even the most feeble minded may be
able to regulate their habits so as to secure an
adequate supply of food both in quality and
quantity, and the prompt removal of waste
matter, so as to secure that degree of cleanliness
of internal organs essential to escape from bacterial attacks, the mechanism of the body is endowed with instincts that make it automatic in
its action. Such are appetite and taste for food
and drinks; the desire for exercise, rest, and
sleep; the impulse of the organs in an active
state, etc. It is only when these natural
monitors are interfered with that the mechanism begins to fail in its elimination of waste,
and bacteria find the conditions favorable for
their functional activity.

THE second defensive measure is the destruction of the bacteria by means of agents that
will destroy the microörganism before or
after its entrance into the body, but without in-
juring the healthy tissues. There is a great variety of these agents of more or less power, and
they are used in the form of gases, liquids, and
powders, according to conditions existing in in-

dividual cases. In general, it may be advised
that, as bacteria are everywhere,
Destroy the   germicides ought to be used far
Bacteria   more extensively than they
are for the purposes of se-
curing not only the direct destruction of bacteria, but of removing or neutralizing dead matter, the food of bacteria.

So minute are bacteria, and so adherent are
they to material things, that mere bathing with
water does not remove them, medicate it as we
may with fancy soaps. There should be used
in addition a more penetrating and destructive
agent, which would not only destroy all forms
of bacteria, but at the same time secure absolute
cleanliness.

IT would be impossible even to summarize, except in a volume, the vast number of so-called
germicides that have been brought to the attention of the public for use; but in the practice
of surgery the chief reliance is placed upon
those agents which simply oxi-
The Value of   dize organic matter, and thus
Germicides   destroy the germ without injur-
ing living tissue, as do all forms
of caustic preparations. The saving of life by
these new measures far exceeds that effected by
simply removing the material that contains the
germ, without destroying the germ itself.

It is impossible to estimate the resources of

science in its efforts to discover the ultimate
conditions that govern the origin and spread of
all the pestilential diseases; but its revelations
during the last quarter of a century are a
prophecy and a promise that the whole brood
of domestic contagious and infectious diseases
will disappear during the present century from
the homes of English-speaking people; largely
because the lessons of cleanliness are being
learned, not only the lessons of cleanliness of
the home, but also personal cleanliness — a
form of cleanliness that is more than washing
with soap and water, — that kind of cleanliness
which kills germs, removes the substances in
which they live, and disinfects and makes
aseptic and healthy the surrounding tissues.

VIII
A Closing Word

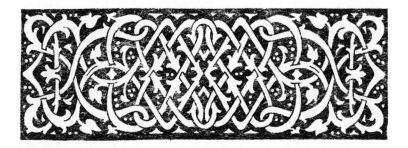

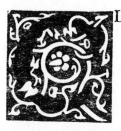"LEANLINESS is indeed next to Godliness," is an oft-quoted saying of John Wesley. Bacon stated the maxim thus: "Cleanness of body was ever deemed to proceed from a due reverence to God." The Hebrew Fathers, from whom this sanitary principle was derived, resolved the doctrines of religion into "Carefulness; Carefulness into Vigor-

Cleanliness Next ousness; Vigorousness into
to Godliness Guiltlessness; Guiltlessness into Abstemiousness; Abstemiousness into Cleanliness; Cleanliness into Godliness."

This religious creed was doubtless based on the Mosaic sanitary code, and was the preventive measure against pestilences which the great Jewish law-giver approved. How generally and how long the "Chosen People" adopted and practised this method of protection against epidemic diseases does not appear, but it is quite certain that in later days it had been discarded.

THE Hebrew Fathers could have had no conception of the invisible agencies in filth that
made uncleanness such a powerful factor in
the propogation of epidemic pestilences and
domestic contagious and infectious diseases. It
was reserved for the scien-
Invisible Agencies   tists of the recent past to
in Filth   discover the exact nature
of the infective germs of
communicable diseases, their origin, their development, their modes of infection; in other
words, their life history.

This discovery revealed the fact that filth in
every form, whether in the rubbish-heap, the
toilet, the garbage, the dust of the floor, or even
in the folds of the hands and feet, the secretions
of the skin and glands, is a culture bed for germ-
producing diseases. The secret of the great
power of cleanness as the true remedial measure for the prevention of pestilences is now apparent and every citizen must recognize that the
obligation of applying that remedy rests with
himself.

The Great Awakening, in the middle of the
last century, of the people of England, and subsequently, of this country, to the intimate relations of filth, in all forms in and around their
dwellings, to the prevalence and fatality of
cholera, typhus fever, and other communicable
diseases, has restored cleanliness to its ancient
imperial position as chief of the virtues, and

the most reliable private and public means of conserving health.

THIS awakening, due both in England and America to trivial incidents, forms one of the most interesting chapters in human history. Already the outcome has been an enormous reduction of the mortality of English-speaking peoples, an immense increase in the length of life, and an advance in the arts of living, which insures a higher civilization by securing to every citizen a sound mind in a sound body.

A Higher Civilization

DOCUMENTS

RELATING TO

The Board of Health.

―――――――――――

NEW-YORK:

PRINTED BY JAMES CHEETHAM,

No. 81, *Pearl-Street.*

1806.

Documents

THE BOARD OF HEALTH.

OFFICE OF THE BOARD OF HEALTH.
NOVEMBER 13, 1805.

TO THE PUBLIC.

ON the termination of their duties of the late calamitous season, the Board of Health consider it no more than a becoming mark of respect to their fellow-citizens, to lay before them such facts as may illustrate the extent of the distress that has so recently interested the sensibility, and affected, in a greater or less degree, the interests of all descriptions of the community.

It is a subject of deep regret, that a collision of opinion exists, not only with respect to the origin, but also in relation to the nature of the malignant disease commonly denominated the Yellow Fever.—While, on the one hand, it is contended that it is imported from abroad, and that it is propagated by contagion, it is on the other hand asserted with equal earnestness, that it originates at home, or is generated on board of vessels, which arrive amongst us, and that it is entirely non-contagious. These discordant opinions, maintained by medical gentlemen of the first respectability and eminence, and which enter deeply into the passions as well as the interests of the community, must necessarily have an inauspicious influence upon most of the leading measures, either of prevention or remedy, adopted by the guardians of the public health.

The partizans of the opposite theories, animated by the heat of debate, and impelled by their different views of the public good, will naturally approve or censure the measures proposed to avert or alleviate this overwhelming calamity, in proportion as they corroborate or militate against their favourite opinions. Although a man possessed of correct views, will proceed in the direct path of duty without being deterred by censure ; still it cannot be controverted, that the support and approbation of an intelligent public, must animate and encourage his exertions. It is not to be denied, that with the most upright intentions, and with the most firm determination, to maintain an impartial official position in the conflict arising from these theories, yet that our conduct may sometimes, insensibly and unintentionally, notwithstanding our utmost circumspection, deviate from the strict line of impartiality. That the inconveniences here stated have in some measure been felt and observed, is highly probable ; but we are happy to note that we have received a candid and honourable support from our fellow-citizens in general, and composed as the Board is of persons holding different tenets, yet that our proceedings have been governed by a spirit of harmony rarely manifested in public bodies.

The importance of exploring every source of correct information, and the expediency of dispassionate and ample deliberation, before an official declaration of the prevalence of malignant fever, must be obvious to all. The universal alarm excited by the existence of this disease, the serious injury to the commercial and agricultural interests of the community, and the extreme inconvenience to our fellow-citizens in particular, render it necessary that the evil should absolutely prevail before it is acknowledged. On the other hand, it is due to the health as well as the security of the lives of our citizens, to apprize them seasonably of the calamity, which menaces them. Circumstanced as the Board were at the commencement of the late malignant disease, well aware that many of their fellow-citizens regarded the few cases which, at that period, had occurred merely as the common bilious fever of the country; sensible of the calamitous consequences which, in either case, would result, of announcing the prevalence of the fever, if it really did not exist, or of not avowing it, if it did; anxious to unite public opinion on a question so deeply interesting, and with the greatest deference and respect to the opinion of the medical gentlemen their associates, who early, uniformly and decidedly declared the evidence of malignant fever, and the probability and danger of an impending pestilential epidemic, the Board considered it their duty to avail themselves of the observations and intelligence of professional gentlemen of different sentiments. Measures were accordingly adopted to obtain their information, and the result was an admission on all sides of the existence of malignant fever.

Although our health laws, in enforcing internal cleanliness, and in subjecting vessels entering our ports to examination, proceed upon the ground that the disease may be either of foreign or domestic origin, yet it is evident they recognize, in common with the health laws of other countries, the doctrine of contagion. Under this impression, the Commissioners of the Health-Office have been authorised, almost since their first establishment, to send all persons and things infected by, or tainted with pestilential matter, to the marine hospital at Staten-Island. By an act of last session, this Board was created, and the Legislature, sensible that the exercise of the power of removal, in this restricted form, would be, in some cases, extremely inconvenient and in others highly pernicious, invested the Board with authority to remove either to the marine hospital or elsewhere. The Board and the Commissioners of the Health-Office have, consequently, a concurrent right to send infected persons and things to the marine hospital, and the Board, moreover, have an exclusive authority to remove them to other places. When some solitary cases occurred, the Board, with a view to arrest the progress of the disease, exercised this discretionary power, but only with the consent of the parties concerned. Afterwards, however, when it was ascertained that the disease was too firmly rooted, to be eradicated by the removal of the sick, the Board considered it their duty to discontinue the application of a remedy, at all times extremely irksome and afflicting, and which perhaps ought only to be resorted to in extreme cases. To the voluntary removal of the healthy from the infected parts of the city, the Board, in a great degree, ascribe the comparative fewness of deaths which have occurred. In the expediency of this step all parties concurred. Whether the disease was communicated by the principle of contagion, or by the influence of an impure atmosphere, the danger was equally alarming, and it was equally expedient to withdraw from it.

From the commencement to the final extinction of the late prevailing disease *six hundred* Cases of Malignant Fever have been reported to the Board. *Two hundred and sixty-two* Deaths as published in the daily bulletins, including those that happened since their discontinuance, have occurred. *Sixty-four* patients, moreover, were sent to the Marine Hospital, *twenty-eight* of whom died of malignant fever. The total number of patients admitted into Bellevue Hospital was *one hundred and seventy-five, one hundred and forty-nine* of which were cases of malignant fever, and *twenty-six* of other diseases. The total number of deaths at the Hospital which were included in the bulletins, was *sixty-nine, fifty-two* of which were by malignant fever, and the remaining *seventeen* by other maladies. The ratio of recoveries from malignant fever is very nearly *two-thirds*, which, considering that a very large proportion of the patients were received in the last stages of disease, and many of them in the very article of death, reflects the highest credit on the practice of the visiting and resident physicians of that establishment.

To alleviate, as far as possible the miseries of the indigent, deprived of all resource for their daily support by the general abandonment of the city, the doors of the Alms-House were opened and rations issued to *sixteen hundred and forty* families. An asylum was erected on the public grounds adjoining Bellevue gate, for the reception of such poor families as the Board judged it expedient to remove from the seat of disease. Every accommodation was afforded to *one hundred and fifty* persons, men women and children, who were maintained by the public bounty. Of this number *thirty* men were daily employed in improving the middle road, leading through the property belonging to the corporation, whose wages tended to lessen the expence incurred by the support of their families. To improve the minds of the children in the asylum, as well as to preserve order and prevent them from becoming obnoxious to the neighbourhood, a school was opened, which afforded instruction, for the space of six weeks, to *forty.* On the propriety and good conduct of this part of the establishment, the Board will long reflect with grateful complacency.

These various objects, combined with the augmentation of the city watch, necessarily involved the Board in an expenditure of *nearly twenty five thousand dollars*, to which it is confidently trusted their fellow citizens will submit with that magnanimity, which has so peculiarly characterized them, on all similar occasions. Excepting the solitary contributions from Boston and Richmond, in Virginia, already acknowledged, amounting to *two hundred and fifty dollars,** the Board have received no eleemosynary aid tow-

* Of the sum here alluded to, two hundred dollars were transmitted from Messieurs James and J. H. Perkins, of Boston, by the hands of Messieurs Grant Forbes and Co. of this city; the other fifty dollars were received from a gentleman in Richmond, Virginia, by the hands of Messieurs Bailey and Bogert.

ards the public exigencies. Voluntary assistance not being proffered, they did not conceive it just to call on their fellow citizens individually—most of whom had to struggle with all the inconveniencies and losses attending removal and the consequent derangement of the regular course of business.

The meetings of the common council being only weekly, the peculiar situation of the city, from its exposure to fire and robbery, in consequence of the evacuation by its inhabitants, rendered it expedient to invest the Board of Health, whose meetings were daily, with a superintending and controlling power over the watchmen and firemen. The board of course paid the utmost attention to these departments, and it is a circumstance of peculiar felicitation, a fact highly honourable to the character of our city, that not a single fire, burglary or robbery, of any consequence, has happened.

To the fidelity and good conduct of the officers of the watch and watchmen, to the care and precaution of the chief engineer, and the indefatigabe vigilence and attention of the special justices of police, the Board deem it their duty to make the most ample acknowledgments. Nor can they omit to mention, in terms of the highest approbation, the unremitted attention of the city inspector in arranging the business and executing the orders of the Board, in all its multifarious details—of the superintendant and commissioners of the Alms-House, in alleviating the distress and administering to the wants of the poor and afflicted— of the medical gentlemen attached to and employed by the Board, who spared no exertions and who shrunk from no danger, in the discharge of their hazardous duties—and generally of the officers of the city and persons in public employment, with whom the Board had official connection, with scarcely a single exception.

The Board will on a future occasion, submit to the proper authority, such measures, as, in their opinion, may appear necessary to be adopted, in order to prevent as far as human means extend, a recurrence of the calamity recently experienced. In the mean time they earnestly solicit a free communication of the sentiments of their fellow citizens on this interesting subject. The Board would do injustice to their feelings, did they not, on this occasion, recommend in the most earnest manner, the destitute widows and orphans of the deceased, to the special benevolence and protection of their fellow citizens. Nor can they omit, in this public manner, to offer up the incense of grateful hearts to the Sovereign Ruler of the Universe, in whose hands are the issues of life and death, for the manifestation of his divine mercy and goodness, in preserving their health and lives amidst surrounding scenes of disease and mortality.

By order, and in behalf of the Board.

DE WITT CLINTON, Pres.

JAMES HARDIE, Sec'ry.

B

THE CITY INSPECTOR'S

𝕽𝖊𝖕𝖔𝖗𝖙.

————— ❊ —————

THE City-Inspector has the honour to report, that in conformity with the wishes of the Board of Health, Bellevue Hospital was finally closed on Saturday, the 28th of October. From its opening on the 9th of September to that day, the number of patients admitted amounted to   175
Of whom the malignant cases were   149
Other diseases,   28

        ——   175

The deaths, which occurred, were as follows:

Of malignant fever, ...	52
typhus fever, ...	3
dysentery, ... ·	3
diarrhœa, ...	3
pneumonia, ...	1
phthysis pulmonalis, . . .	1
epilepsy, . . : . . .	3
cholera infantum, ...	1
diseases unknown, ...	2

                     79
Discharged cured. 106

            Total,   175

The Physicians of the hospital remark, that only ONE

person died, who was admitted on the first day of disease. Four of the patients were, on closing the hospital, sent to the city hospital, cured of fever, but convalescent from chronic diseases.

Of the extreme cases died

within 24 hours after admission, ...	5
12 hours, ...	6
6 hours, ...	3
1 hour, ...	6
10 minutes, ...	2
	22

nearly one-third of the total amount of deaths.

The ratio of cures from malignant fever to deaths by the same disorder is very nearly two thirds. which, considering that most of the patients were sent there in the last stage of disease and death, reflects the highest credit on the practice of Doctors Walker and Winfield, the visiting and resident physicians.

Accompanying this report is the return of the physicians, with the list of patients admitted into the hospital during the present season, likewise a schedule of the state of the hospital for the year 1803 ; by which it appears, that the hospital on that occasion was opened on the 12th day of August, and closed on the 7th of November, during which period were admitted

Of malignant fever patients,		170
Of various other diseases,		21
	Total,	191

The deaths which occurred were,

Of malignant fever, ...	100	
phthysis pulmonalis, . . .	1	
diarrhœa, ...	2	
	130	
Discharged cured, ...	88	

Of whom were sent to the City Hospital,   3
         to the Alms-House,   10
                          —
                        13

on the 7th of November, when the hospital was closed.

A comparative view of these tables shows, that the present season, although nearly one month shorter, has been proportionably more active, and that the success attending the practice of the hospital has been greater this season than the former : as the number of deaths in 1803 considerably exceeded one-half of the cases, and, as before remarked, during the current year, amounted only to about one-third.

The City Inspector wishes it to be understood, that the comparison is made from no invidious motive, and without the most remote idea of reflection on the former services at the hospital, but solely for the satisfaction of the Board, and to furnish data for reflection and calculation, whether the treatment of this awful malady is not better understood, and that a reasonable hope may be entertained, that at no distant day it will be divested of its horrors, and become more controllable and less mortal, by the skill and experience of medical professors.

By the return from the Marine Hospital it appears, that from the 18th day of July to the 28th of October, the number of patients sent from this city, amounted to   64
  Of whom died of malignant fever,   .   28
  Discharged cured, ...   30
  Remained of chronic complaints,   •   6
                              —

               Total,   64

The total number of cases reported at the Office from the 5th of September to the 25th of October inclusive, amounted to   600

The total number of deaths which occurred in this city and at Bellevue Hospital during the same period, as published in the daily bulletins, was   249

To which are to be added the deaths that have
happened since the reports were closed, and
which have been announced in the bills of
mortality amounting to   . .   13

                                  ——— 262

Making in all, 262 deaths of malignant fever.

The total number of cases reported in 1803 appears to
have been 1639.

The deaths by malignant fever, which occurred the same
year, amounted to 606.

In closing his official report for the present season, the
City-Inspector begs leave to submit a few remarks respecting the establishment at Bellevue—the result of his observations and experience.

The buildings called hospitals erected at Bellevue appear
to have been set up on the spur of the occasion, and on the
presumption that the fever would never recur again. Fatal
experience has proved otherwise, and points to the convic_
tion that we may expect repeated attacks from this insidious disease. The wards, the one appropriated for the men
especially, are every way inadequate to the wants of the
patients or the comfort of the nurses and physicians. The
buildings are on too contracted a scale—of materials too
slight to repel the summer heat or autumnal cold. The
crouded state of the hospital, during the last season, must
have had an unfavourable influence on the spirits of the patients. Those newly arrived were evidently depressed by
the surrounding scenes of malady, and the groans and
shrieks of convulsed and dying subjects. The senses were
evidently offended, and the atmostphere rendered impure
in consequence of the wards being so overcrouded. More
extensive accommodations are absolutely necessary against
another season; which it is confidently trusted that the
Board will, at all events, provide.

To render this establishment more extensively useful
and to relieve such persons as may be in ciscumstances to

14

pay for comfortable accommodations, a pay hospital, with suitable distinct apartments, might be advantageously erected. The difficulty of providing for strangers and single gentlemen, labouring under malignant fever, in private families, has been sensibly experienced—such persons are competent and willing to pay liberally for genteel accommodations, were such provided, and there is no doubt that such a branch of the establishment, if not productive, would at least not become burthensome, and would be highly creditable to our city.

Perhaps in regarding the proposed improvements at Bellevue Hospital, it might be of moment to consider, whether a change of the establishment to some other ground appertaining to the Corporation, would not be eligible. The scite of Bellevue might, in all probability, be sold for a sum adequate to very extensive improvements. The accommodation of poor families in suitable buildings, is a part of the whole establishment, which will also deserve the contemplation of the Board, and it is submitted whether the present assylum ought not to be preserved until more permanent buildings can be provided.

All which is respectfully submitted.

JOHN PINTARD, City-Inspector.

New-York, 12th Nov, 1805.

A LETTER FROM

THE HEALTH OFFICER

To The Board of Health.

A LETTER

FROM

THE HEALTH OFFICER

TO

THE BOARD OF HEALTH.

THE HON. DE WITT CLINTON, PRESIDENT, AND THE MEM-
BERS OF THE BOARD OF HEALTH.

New-York, December 19, 1805.

GENTLEMEN,

The late melancholy distress of our city while it has called up the feelings of humanity has excited the public attention to the probable causes of the calamity—this subject has
frequently exercised the judgments of many, and while a
contrariety of opinions has been held, the laws endeavour-
ing to provide against such evils have always supposed that
internal causes as well as *external*, frequently produced the
terrible effect. Your wishes and request, which I respect,
and a desire that the public may know as much on this subject as they can, have induced me to state such facts as will
show, *that whatever may have been the cause of our late epidemic, it did not arise from any neglect in the performance of
duty at the quarantine-ground, nor did it come through that
channel.* I perform this service the more readily, because with the attempts to prove the importation of the disease, private insinuations are made and listened to, injurious to the health department, and designed to operate
against me.

When a law enjoins the performance of certain duties,
and prescribes the line of conduct of the public officers un-

C

der it, if they punctually perform all these injunctions, and faithfully fulfil all their duties—if they extend the performance of the letter so as even to reach the spirit of the law— if they do more than is necessary to secure the former, that cavillers themselves may be satisfied, then are they entirely vindicated to their own consciences, and to the public— and even if the law should be utterly insufficient to accomplish the objects proposed, still are they completely justified.

The candid enquirer after truth in this case will distinguish between the law and the officer, and he will never blend the two together.

The exclusive importers, who reject all internal causes of disease, ought also to look at the different quarters by which it may, according to their judgment and theory, invade us —they ought to advert to the chances of bringing disease in foul clothes, and by the persons of men, from other places, as well as the Quarantine Ground—if disease can come from infected places abroad, and at a distance, it assuredly can come from like places at home, and close at our doors—New-Haven, Providence, and Philadelphia had the disease as soon as, and perhaps before, New-York. —The communication between these places and our city was open and constant, and the access easy—Why not bring it from them, as well as from the Quarantine-Ground? The danger of bringing disease from those places, is acknowledged, by the Board of Health taking measures to cut off the communication between them and New-York. These measures were strictly attended to on the sea board, but I am not so certain that they were attended to on the land side. Candid people, who hold to the theory of exclusive importation, acknowledge the force of these observations, but others, not so just, are anxious to bring the disease only by the Quarantine Ground, the better to establish a particular point of theory, and perhaps to injure the Health Officer.

As attempts have been made by some to prejudice the public mind against me, because I believe in other causes of disease than importation, I hold it right here to say, that I consider myself merely an executive officer, and whatever the law directs, I have ever, and shall ever perform, to the best of my ability, with fidelity and care. As an officer, I obey the law in all its prescriptions, without examining its merits or demeri s.

I believe, as I have ever declared, in the propriety of cleansing foul ships—of purifying and changing bad air, and of preventing impure materials or diseased persons from going up to a large city. But I believe too, that diseases originate at home, when they are often looked for from abroad and this I believe in my conscience was the case last season. But to show, that whatever was the cause of the disease or wherever it may have arisen, it did not come through the Quarantine Ground; let us attend to the following facts.---

No vessel from a place where pestilential fever prevailed at the time of her departure, or where the place was supposed sickly, has approached the city of New-York, nearer than the quarantine ground, from the first of June to the first of October; nor has any vessel, on board of which any person has died with pestilential or any other fever, from the West-Indies or any other part interdicted by law, or been sick with the same, gone up to the city of New-York this whole season—no sick person, of any description, has been suffered to go into the city of New-York, through the summer or autumn, except one person, an invalid and with a chronic complaint, and who had been in the marine hospital a month before he left us.

No foul materials, dirty clothes, or articles interdicted by law, have gone beyond the public store at the quarantine ground, from the first of June to the first of October—nor has any of the officers, seamen, or passengers belonging to, or arriving in the vessels which have been detained at quarantine, had malignant fever, except in one single instance, about the 12th of September, as I shall state in another place. *Nor can any of the cases of fever which have occurred in the city, be traced to any of the vessels kept at quarantine, or to any other vessel, or person, or thing, which has passed through our hands.* Of the many seamen and passengers who had arrived from the West-Indies, and other ports subject to quarantine of course, and indeed all foreign ports, not one was seized with malignant fever before the 30th of August, and not till after the disease had been decidedly in the city forty-two days, and not till after *seven* persons (citizens) had been sent from New-York to the marine hospital with the complaint—and excepting *this individual*, not one of those who came to us had been for many months before, either in the West-Indies, or on board of any infected vessel.

At the quarantine ground there have been constantly from the first of June to the first of October, a considerable number of vessels; frequently during that time, from forty to fifty, and on the last day of September, sixty—All of these vessels had either lost some one or more of their crews, or had come from a sickly port; many of them (twenty-four in number) were under the necessity of coming to the public wharf, where some of them lay the greater part of the season; one vessel 106 days, another 44 days, and a third 38, a fourth 37, and so on—Of these, a considerable number hove down, others threw out their ballast, or cleansed their limbers; some were sheathed or graved, and all of them overhauled more or less; and of the many officers, seamen, and workmen, ship-carpenters, caulkers, riggers, coopers, sail-makers, blacksmiths, &c. not one was in the smallest degree indisposed, or took any sickness by connection with those vessels; nor has any of these persons that I know of, been indisposed, except one carpenter, who took sick some weeks after he left the quarantine ground, and died in the latter part of September in New-York; having exposed himself in the poisoned air of the city. Of the pilots who have brought these infected vessels into port, and had frequently slept on board of them, very often one night and sometimes two, before they came to at quarantine, not one (or any of their families,) has been in the smallest degree indisposed from any connection with such vessel. Of those attached to the Health-Officer's department, boatmen, orderlies, nurses, washerwomen and attendants, not one has been sick from any infection, or from any connection with the sick or infected vessels. Of the lighterers employed in carrying goods to the city, or bringing cargoes to vessels at quarantine, not one was in the smallest degree indisposed till the 24th or 25th of September, when one of them was taken with fever, which left him in a few days—Another was seized just after the first, and died the 2d of October. Neither of these had had any connection with any foul ship to which they could attribute their complaint; but they took it from having had a daily intercourse with the eastern part of the city, and from being under the necessity of going into houses and stores in that quarter, and staying longer in them than they had been accustomed to, by reason of the want of hands to receive their goods, in consequence of the desertion of that part of the city.

The masters of vessels, passengers, and seamen, with their baggage, going from the quarantine ground, pass in one or two particular boats, and land at the Whitehall wharf, and almost all the sick people sent to the marine hospital from the city, embark at that slip, and yet none of the persons going or passing in these boats, or conveying these sick, have been in the slightest degree indisposed; nor was there a single case of fever in the neighbourhood of the Whitehall, till the 19th of September, and long after it had appeared in several other parts of the city, distant from that quarter. The first case of malignant or yellow fever which came from on board of a vessel at the time of her arrival at quarantine, was on the 12th of September; all the other cases of fever which had come from on board ship before, were of the remitting type, were freed from the strong symptoms marking yellow fever, and in a day or two after admission, assumed the intermitting form, and were all cured by the bark. The sickliest vessels which have arrived this season, have been from our own country, and had no intercourse with West-Indian or other supposed infected ports. From these facts, you will see that no injury has been suffered by any infection coming into port, and operating upon those who are below the city ; nor has any arisen in the track of communication between the quarantine and the city, or from the communication itself, in any form, or in any place. If it had arisen from the communication, it would have appeared first, and most, among people on that track ; among those *going to*, or *residing at* Whitehall—but the fact is directly the reverse ; the people on that route have been altogether well, and that neighbourhood was the last to suffer, notwithstanding the number of sick brought to it, on their way to the quarantine ground.

I shall now relate the names and dates of admission of the different patients with malignant fever, and the places from which they came. I go into this detail, that you may judge whether the disease went from the quarantine ground to New-York, or came from the city to us. Although there is good reason to suppose that the disease in question was in the city before the beginning of July, and though from the testimony of others I believe it, yet from my situation on Staten-Island, I can only speak of what I there saw, and what came to us. It admits, however, of no controversy, that the persons from Maiden-lane in July, had malignant fever, and four people were in succession seized with the same symptoms, and came at different times with the same complaint. These men had no connection with shipping, and it was denied by those who had not seen them, that their complaint was malignant fever, because it could not be traced to any vessel; but to deny the truth of a position or fact, because it does not agree with our theory, is to shut the door at once on reasoning.

All those who did see these men, agree that their disease was malignant fever, and those who did not see them, cannot be so competent to decide. The two first who came from Maiden-lane, were *Christopher Hibborn* and *William Aylsbury*—They arrived on the 18th of July—On the 30th of July *Mr. Dougherty* was admitted; he came from Water-street, between the Coffee-House and Pine-street. This man was readily acknowledged to have malignant fever, because it was expected to trace it to shipping—it was said. he had intercourse with an Irish ship at quarantine ; there is however no proof of this, and the strong probability is that he had not, as well from the affidavits which have been taken, as from the declarations of the officers and men to that purpose—and even if he had intercourse with the ship, he could have gotten no disease from her, for she was healthy—had been so during the whole voyage—came from an healthy port in Ireland, and all the passengers and people have continued healthy to this day, as far as I know—during Dougherty's supposed visit or visits to the quarantine ground, no one was sick with fever, either in the quarantine road, or the hospital, nor had any one been yet sick with this complaint in either of these places, for it was before the time that Hibborn and Aylesbury were admitted— But Dougherty had no direct or personal communication with any vessel at quarantine.

On the 7th of August, *Isabella Adams*, from Chamber-street, was admitted with malignant fever. No intercourse with shipping has ever been intimated in her case. August 16th *Mrs. Phyfer*, from Water street the next door to the corner of Wall street, came down. She had been ill five or six days before her admission. She had no connection with shipping, or any intercourse with any person or thing from any ship. August 20, *Jamas Laughan*, from Maiden-Lane, and on the 23d, *Andrew Stayley* from the same place, came to us. Here then are *seven* persons from the City, admitted with fever, before a single sailor has even *sickened* with the complaint. On the 30th of August, *Joshua Haines, a seaman*, was admitted; he had been in port since the 15th of August, had arrived in an healthy vessel from an healthy port, and did not arrive till after several persons had sickened and died with fever, both in the city, and at the marine hospital. On the 1st and 2d of September, *Alfred Preston* and *William Frazer*, house-carpenters, were admitted—the one resided in *Division* and the other in *Chapple* streets; both of them had worked at the same time at the new houses at and near the corner of Wall and Water streets, neither of them had had any intercourse whatever with either ships or seamen.— On the 3d *David Pymer, his wife* and *two children* were admitted; all of these were but slightly affected, except one of the children, who died with malignant fever; they came from the lower end of Pine-street. On the 4th, *Jacob Christopher*, a seaman from on board the brig Columbia, from Boston, lying in the Coffee-House-slip. On the 6th, *Charles Everitt, labourer*, from the Bear-Market.—On the 7th *Matthew Burke*, seaman, from the schooner Eliza, coaster; *Richard Thompson*, labourer, from Front-street, and *Ann Brady*, from Depeyster-street. On the 8th, *Charles Diven*, labourer, from Elm-street, *Eustace Long*, labourer, Rider-street, *Henry Blackman*, Pearl-street, *Mrs. Beekman*, foot of Wall-street, and *Richard H. Midge*, seaman, from the schooner Weymouth, a coasting vessel, at a wharf on the North River. 9th, *Stephen Fenlar*, Fly-market. 10th, *Jonathan Campbell*, Pine-street. 12th, *Daniel Cox* and *John Haidley*, seamen, from the ship Flora, at Gaine's wharf. On the 15th, *James Keaugh* and *Richard Adams*, from the corner of Pine and Front streets. On the 16th, *John Marino*, seaman, from the ship Delaware, from Hull, at Rector-street wharf; 20th, *James Develine* and *child*, from corner of Pine and Front streets; 23d, *Samuel*

Munkley, from the ship Selemo, from New-York, outward bound. 24th, *Robert Davis*, labourer, Pine-street, and *Charles Fanning*, Fly-market. 25th, *Daniel Burton*, labourer, Depeyster-street, *Charles Corvel*, labourer, Georges's-street wharf, and *Mrs. Develine*, corner of Pine and Front streets. 30th of September, *William Bonant*, labourer, James-street, and *Leonard Doven*, labourer, from James-street. On the 2d of October, *John Lawson*, labourer, from James-street, was admitted ; the 5th, *John Tindle*, from the Fly-market ; 9th, *William Logard*, labourer, from New-York, place of abode not known ; 15th, *Thomas Smith*, seaman, from the ship Earl of Lansdale, arrived within a fortnight from the West-Indies : 28th of October, *Thomas Ha。milton*, from Water-street, labourer.

You have in this detail *forty-five* patients—of these *ten* were seamen ; and of these ten, but three had been in the West-Indies, or had had any intercourse with any foreign port, from which malignant fever is supposed to come—of these three, *one* arrived in August, from an healthy port, in an healthy vessel, and not till after several had died with yellow fever ; one came into port, and was immediately taken into the hospital, and the *other* arrived in the latter end of October—No one will for a moment suppose that either of these introduced or propagated yellow fever.—Of the remaining *thirty-five*, *three* were *women*, *three children*, and *twenty-nine men ;*—of these last, *twelve* were labourers, the greater part, if not all, having been at sea,*but *none of them within several months previous to their coming into the marine hospital, and none of them having the smallest idea, of having contracted the disease, by any intercourse with any person, or thing coming from on board a vessel, or from abroad.*—You will observe that the first fifteen persons sent down (with the exception of *Isabella Adams* and *Joshua Haines*) were from Maiden-lane, and a particular neighbourhood in Water-street ; which neighbourhood did not exceed two hundred yards from the one extremity to the

26

other. The circumstance of so many sickening in one house and within so narrow a compass in Water-street, and the disease having appeared in a former year *first* in that very neighbourhood, and in every year of pestilence, *always* first shewing itself in situations precisely similar, establish the position of a domestic origin. Nor can it be pretended that the communication between the quarantine could produce it *here*, because this was exactly the place where, of all others, the communication was the least, nay there could be none at all, for there were no stores directly behind where Mrs. *Phyfer* and *Frazer* and *Preston* took sick. Nor had any of these 35 patients been at the quarantine* at any time of the summer previous to their admission, nor had any of them any connection with infected ships or diseased persons. You see then that West-India vessels did not produce it, for but *one West-India* vessel had but *one* sick with malignant fever, while *three coasters* and *two European* vessels sent down *seven* patients. You see from this statement, and from the experience of this season, that *ships* have been freer from disease than *houses* ; that *seamen* have been incomparably healthier than *citizens;* and that the W. India vessels sent up from quarantine, have been less infected than our own coasters—does this prove that the evil came from the quarantine ground? Let candor judge.— Had it arisen from West-India vessels, it must have appeared sooner on the Long-Island shore, where there were more of these vessels, than in the East river, and as soon in the North river, where nearly as many lay as on the East side of the city. Had the infection extended itself from these, or other vessels in the East river, then the persons on board of the vessels along side the wharf, the cartmen working on the quays, and the merchants and their clerks in the stores in South-street, would have been first seized, and in succession, as the poison passed along ; but none of these

---

* Unless you except Dougherty.

were affected at all. The line along the river was healthy till you approached the evils which were entrenched a little farther in. Then you came to the seat of pestilence; and when you consider the nature of the occupations of all those who sickened and died from Wall-street to the Fly-market in Pearl-street, and those who sickened in Water-street, you will not attach blame to ships.

It will not do to say that the air was bad, and thus was the conductor to some evil secretly introduced; for this is giving up almost the whole of the question. How came this air so bad? How came it more vitiated and within so small a compass? If it were bad sooner in Water-street, than in Front, and still much sooner than in South-street, it must have arisen from other causes than shipping; it must have arisen from the influence of the atmosphere on local impurities---and no one can point to the person or thing bringing this evil to *that* neighbourhood.

I shall now consider the only rumour that has any thing like a specific form; it is what you have on your files, and given on the 6th of September, stating, " that Patrick Ben-
" son, who is a dealer in rigging, went frequently to the
" quarantine ground, and as Benson told the deponent, two
" or three times a week for the purpose of buying rigging,
" sails, &c. and brought them to the city; that the depo-
" nent lives at 132 Front-street, and Benson in the cellar of
" the same house; that about two or three weeks ago (the
" information being given Sept. 6th) Benson brought up at
" least two cart loads of rigging, &c. old sails, and old coats,
" and deposited them in the cellar of that house, and that
" Benson took sick yesterday (Sept. 5) but is better this
" morning; that the deponent has seen great numbers of
" working men go down, as they said, to the quarantine
" ground and return as riggers and stevadores from Mr.
" Englis who keeps a boarding-house at the foot of Pine
" and Front-streets."

It is intended by this vague statement, to convey an insinuation that the quarantine communication being too open, permitted dirty old clothes to come up and that they made Patrick Benson, and perhaps others, sick. Let us hear what Patrick Benson himself says. " Patrick Benson, dealer in rigging, &c. being duly sworn deposeth and saith, that he has been employed in buying old junk and rigging for some months past, and that he always bought the same at, and in the city of New-York, and never on board of vessels in the stream, or from along side of the wharf. The deponent further saith that he never went to the quarantine ground for the purpose of buying rigging but once, and that at this particular time he did not buy any thing, but only inspected some old junk on the public wharf in the presence of the officer of the customs, not being able to agree with the owner in the price. That this deponent afterwards bought this same junk from a man who had sent it to the White-hall, which man had, as he was told, a regular permit from the custom-house to inspect the same. That the above deponent was several times at the different ferries at each side of the quarantine ground during the summer, but that he never went inside of the quarantine ground, without a regular permit from the health officer. That he was permitted to work on board of vessels after he left the city in September, and never before, and that after this time he did not return to the city but twice 'till the fever had disappeared, and at each time he had permission to come up. The deponent further saith that he never was on board of any vessel at quarantine, for any purpose whatever, before the 6th of September, and that he never knew or heard of any person holding intercourse with ships or the quarantine ground, but by the permission of the health officer. The said deponent further saith, that all his family were well during the whole season, excepting himself, who was, from fatigue, indisposed on the evening of the 5th of September, but, on taking a vomit, was entirely relieved, so as to go to work on the 6th, and to remove to Staten-Island on the 7th. The said deponent further saith, that he never bought any clothes of any description at the quarantine ground, or old clothes, elsewhere, within two years last past."

his

PATRICK ⋈ BENSON.

mark.

Sworn 11*th Dec.* 1805,⎱
before Dewitt Clinton. ⎰   (Copy.)

But riggers and stevedores, it is said, *went without permission to the quarantine ground.* This is denied. They never entered the quarantine ground without permission. They might have gone whenever they pleased, to either of the ferries on each side of the quarantine ground, and no one has the power, or the right to prevent it. They might probably have gone in considerable numbers there, because many hands were absolutely necessary, to enable the merchants to repair, and load their vessels, and these people often returned to the city, not being able to get the enormous wages they wished. But they never entered the quarantine ground, or left it, without permission. And when they had worked on board of infected vessels, they never immediately returned to the city, and not without the master, or employer, or leader of the party, giving security, and being answerable for their return, if necessary. I must remark that the merchants have frequently suffered by the indiscretion of some people in the city, who being entirely ignorant of the arrangements at quarantine, represented every part of the ground and the establishment, and every vessel in the roads, as equally infected and equally dangerous to deal with. They represented the danger of even the atmosphere blowing over one vessel and tainting another. These are the people who have raised the wages of men working at the quarantine ground. None of these men, supposed to have so improperly passed, have either received, or communicated disease. Nor did any captain, or supercargo, or passenger, go from an infected vessel, without being under an obligation, either not to go into the city, or if he were permitted to enter the city, to return within a limitted time : and as no injury has arisen, and no one has violated his obligation, it is fair to conclue that no evil went from the quarantine ground to New-York. It behoves those who assert, or suspect that there was any improper communication, to prove their assertion, or to give the reasons for their suspicion, and more especially what they know, or have heard, respecting any thing of the kind in the night time. If any one believing in the danger arising from a breach of the revenue, or health laws, were to know of such violation, especially in the night time, and were to conceal it from the proper officers, he would be guilty of great neglect of duty to the public, and might almost be esteemed *particeps criminis.* We have happily this season, detected all that infringed the quarantine laws.

This unlimitted communication then did not obtain, for it could not have escaped the strict care and scrutiny of the custom-house and quarantine officers, or the vigilant attention of the board of health.

I must now for a moment advert to the story of rags from Algesiras, against which a prejudice has been raised. It so happens, from the dates of occurrences, that the rags would be clear from any imputation of blame, even if they had been dirty; *but they were clear and perfectly innoxious.* They had been prepared in the way they always are for the psrposes of commerce; that is, after being first washed clean, dipped into, or through a strong lime water, or an alkaline solution; then dried and packed in bags or bales. These rags thus prepared, were shipped some time last sprng from Leghorn, on board of an English vessel for Liverpool or London. The vessel was captured by a Spanish privateer and taken into Algesiras, where the vessel and rags were bought by the agent of Mr. J. Hurtin of this city. The vessel had an health bill from Leghorn, and one also from Algesiras. She arrived here in August, after a passage of fifty-six days of mild weather, during which the hatches were always off in the day time, and the people almost constantly over the bags. The crew was healthy, and had been so during the whole voyage, and the rags dry and in good order. When the bags were ripped open they gave out a white inodorous dust or powder—this powder was lime. These rags were landed on the 13th of August, at the end of Coenties wharf, were there from 8 o'clock in the morning 'till 12 at noon of the same day, and only for the purpose of being weighed ; they were then taken on board a vessel bound to the eastward. A sample bag had been at Mr. Hurtin's store, two days previously to landing the rest, and was then taken, away. No person has received any injury from these rags nor possibly could, for they were clean and as inoffensive as any article in the city.

I have now clearly shewn as far as negative proof can go, *that whatever might have been the cause of the late epidemic,* *it did not arise from any neglect of duty at the quarantine* *ground,* NOR DID IT COME THROUGH THAT CHANNEL.

I cannot conclude this communication, gentlemen, without offering my tribute of gratitude and thanks to that Providence which has so happily preserved your lives and health during the late pestilence. May you long be spared as blessings to your country !

With much respect,

I have the honor to be

Your obedient servant,

JOHN R. B. RODGERS.

A LETTER FROM

Dr. *EDWARD MILLER*,

RESIDENT PHYSICIAN,

TO

HIS EXCELLENCY GOVERNOR CLINTON,

DATED

New-York, January 6, 1804.

Sir,

I have been honored with your excellency's letter of the
26th ult. which, by some accident of the post-office, did not
come to my hands, till the day before yesterday. I greatly
regret the delay, which has taken place in transmitting an
account of the late malignant disease in this city; but I rely
on your goodness to excuse it, when you learn that your in-
timation on the subject was the first notice I received, that
either the desire of the governor, or the custom of my pre-
decessors had made such a report a part of my official duty.

The commencement of the disease took place about the
20th of July; and, from that time, it continued to prevail,
in a greater or less degree, till the end of October. The
number of deaths in this city amounted to five hundred and
three; those at the hospital of Bellevue to one hundred
three, and those at the Marine hospital on Staten-Island
to sixty-eight; making a total of six hundred and seventy-
four. To this should be added an indefinite number, about
fifty or sixty, who fled from the city, and died of this disease, in the neighboring country and villages.

The first public alarm arose from some fatal cases, at the
Coffee-house slip, and in that neighborhood. About the
same time, the disease was discovered in many other parts
of the city, without any known intercourse or communication between the persons, who fell sick. Although the number of cases, even at the worst periods of the epidemic,
could never be pronounced to be great, especially if compared with some preceding seasons, they were certainly more
generally diffused and left fewer parts of the city exempt

than on any former occasion. Broadway, and some of the adjacent parts of the town, retained their healthy character. The streets lying near the margins of the two rivers, and some of those in the upper parts of the town, which are principally inhabited by indigent, uncleanly and dissolute classes of the community, suffered the worst ravages of the disease. The alarm of the inhabitants was very suddenly produced ; and the suspension of business and desertion of the city, far exceeded what had been ever experienced in preceding seasons.

As to the source from which this epidemic was derived, your excellency is well acquainted with the diversity of opinions, which still subsists in the United States. The question whether the disease was introduced from abroad, or generated by domestic causes, has been discussed, in no former season, with more animation and inflexibility.

Those, who contend for the foreign origin of the disease, believe in the importation of it, by some vessel, or vessels, which arrived at this port early in July. Three vessels are mentioned, the *Hibbert*, the *Gypsy* and *La Victoire ;* the two former from Europe, and the last from St. Domingo. The particular circumstances of each of these ships, shall be stated in order.

The British ship *Hibbert* arrived from Portsmouth (England) on the 4th July. Every person on board was in perfect health, and had been so during the passage of fifty days. This ship, as it afterwards appeared, contained a great deal of filth, which, for a long time, had been suffered to accumulate, while she was employed in transport-service. Though this filth had remained inoffensive in the mild climate of England, and, likewise, during the voyage (for no sickness had occurred on board) the Hibbert did not lie more than two weeks at Ackerley's wharf, in the very hot weather of July, before she emitted a most noisome smell, and several persons engaged in removing the rubbish and filth from the hold were seized with all the symptoms of yellow fever. This happened about the 10th of July.

The British ship *Gypsy* arrived on the 3d of July, from St. Ubes in Portugal, laden with salt; every person on board was in perfect health. St. Ubes was entirely free from any malignant or epidemic disease at the time of her sailing, which was regularly certified by a bill of health. The Gypsy had no sickness on board, while she lay at St. Ubes, during the voyage thence to New-York, nor until seventeen days after her arrival at this port. All these circumstances are attested under the oath of the captain. After lying seventeen days in this port, she became sickly, and lost a large portion of her hands by the yellow fever.

The French ship *La Victoire*, on which the principal charge of importing yellow fever has been laid, arrived from Cape-Francois on the 12th of July. Every person on board was in perfect health. She had sailed from Dunkirk on the 10th of March; after a voyage of forty-one days, she arrived at Cape-Francois with a cargo of dry goods : she lay at Cape-Francois two months and a few days; and then set sail for New-York, where she arrived at the time before mentioned. During the voyage from Dunkirk to Cape-Francois, during the time she lay in the harbor of Cape-Francois, and during the voyage from the Cape to New-York, no sickness occurred on board, except one case of dysentery at Cape-Francois, which terminated in recovery. The Cape, at that season, was remarkably free from yellow fever ; the bill of health brought by this ship purported that it was entirely so ; and the same was confirmed by a surgeon on board. The cargo consisted of coffee, put up in close casks, sugar and lignumvitæ. She was detained for some days at the quarantine ground, for the purpose of inspecting the coffee, which was found in the best condition. While she lay at the quarantine ground, she was ventilated, white-washed, and the clothes and bedding washed and aired. The day before the permit was given for proceeding to New-York, a block fell from aloft on the head of a sailor, which hurt him considerably, but not so much as to make it expedient to detain him at the Marine hospital. No other sickness had taken place in this vessel up to the 20th of August, when this account was circumstantially delivered under the signature of the captain. All the leading facts now stated had been given by him to the health officer, under oath, at the time of his arrival. I have been the more particular in this account of *La Victoire*, as she was the vessel, on which the charge of importation chiefly, and almost exclusively, has been made to rest.

From these facts, it seems to result, that, if our malignant disease was really introduced from abroad by any of the vessels, charged with having imported it, the introduction must have taken place either from parts of Europe, where the disease did not exist, and in vessels, which had no sickness on board till some time after arrival here, or in a vessel from St. Domingo, on board of which no case of yellow fever had appeared, and which arrived at New-York, under very extraordinary circumstances of health and cleanliness.

The circumstances of the ship *Hibbert*, are important and instructive. They prove, that a foul ship from an English port, where yellow fellow fever is never known, with all the crew and passengers in a perfectly healthy state, may become, after lying some time at one of our wharves in very hot weather, a source of the most malignant disease. And they likewise prove, that filthy vessels, even from the most healthy ports, are often as proper objects of examination, detention and cleansing, as those from the West-Indies.

The different opinions concerning the origin of yellow fever, would seem, on a slight survey of the subject, to lead to very different means of prevention and public safety; but more attentive consideration will impress the opposite conviction. Both parties insist on the necessity of detaining and cleansing foul and sickly vessels; the importers of yellow fever from abroad, for the purpose of excluding contagion—and the advocates of domestic generation, for the purpose of removing that filth, which, by the operation of heat, is so readily converted into poisonous vapour.

As to the removal of nuisances in the city, and rendering it as clean and pure as possible, all parties, even on their own principles, ought to be equally agreed. Yellow fever is known to spread and prevail, in certain seasons, in this city. But it is also known, that, at such times, it cannot spread and prevail in the adjacent country and villages. In every season of this epidemic at New-York, multitudes have fled to the country, to Newark, Elizabeth-Town, Brunswick, &c. where they have been seized with the disease, and have died, without communicating it to any inhabitants of those places. The difference of condition and circumstances between such towns and this city, which, in the one case, annihilates the disease, at the death or recovery of the patient, and in the other, causes it to spread and become epidemic, must entirely consist in the absence of nuisances from the former, and in the accumulation and predominance of them in the latter. It seems, therefore, to follow of course, that the great desideratum towards banishing yellow fever from New-York, however it may be supposed to originate, *is such a degree of cleanliness and purity as may be found in the villages of the neighborhood,* or as near an approximation to it as possible. Such a system of police as this, vigorously adopted and enforced, aided by the regulations of the Health Establishment on Staten-Island, which are most strictly and vigilantly executed, would, in my judgment, completely secure this city from the ravages of the yellow fever.

With sentiments of the highest respect,

I have the honor to be,

Your Excellency's most obedient

and humble servant,

EDWARD MILLER,

Resident Physician.

REPORT

ON

Ehe Malignant Disease,

WHICH PREVAILED IN THE CITY OF NEW-YORK,

IN THE AUTUMN OF 1805:

ADDRESSED TO THE GOVERNOR

OF THE

STATE OF NEW-YORK.

BY EDWARD MILLER, M. D.
Resident Physician for the City of New-York.

F

☞ *DISTANT readers will be better enabled to under-stand this report by adverting to the following particulars. The City of New-York lies in N lat. 40 42 8 ; W. long. 74 9 45 ; at the confluence of the river Hudson and Long-Island sound or the East river ; and on the southern and narrow extremity of Manhattan-Island, which is about* 15 *miles in length, and from one to two in breadth. The site of the City, as it originally stood, was very irregular, being broken into hills and declivities, and indented with small rivulets or creeks, skirted with marsh. Many of the hills are levelled ; but the marshy grounds, though covered with houses and pavement, are still low and moist. The City is about* 27 *miles from the ocean, and is washed on both sides with water of great depth, whose current is very rapid, whose tide ebbs and flows about* 6 *feet, and which is nearly as salt as that of the neighbouring sea. On both sides of the City considerable encroachments have been made on the water by artificial ground, the whole extent of which may be computed at not less than* 132 *acres. Of this,* 90 *acres lie along the East river, and* 42 *along the Hudson. The portion of it on the East river forms that part of the City where malignant fevers have always first become epidemic and chiefly prevailed. The wharves and docks are constructed of logs and loose stones. All the fresh water used by the inhabitants is procured from wells within the City, and is now become extremely impure. The population of New-York may be estimated at about* 80,000.

New-York, Jan. 12*th*, 1806.

SIR,

THE Malignant Disease which prevailed in this city, for
a considerable part of last autumn, having ceased about the
beginning of November, it becomes my duty to lay before
your Excellency such an account of it as my official situation
has enabled me to collect. I undertake this task with the
more readiness, and shall examine the subject with the more
attention, as this disease has lately acquired great additional importance from the frequency of its recurrence, the
extent of its ravages, and the new and alarming points of
view in which it is now considered by the nations of Europe. The embarrassments of our commerce on this account, in foreign ports, have been increasing for several
years; they are already become oppressively great; they are
likely hereafter to become still greater; and nothing but a
thorough investigation of the subject, and the adoption of a
wise and mature system of measures, will be sufficient to
ascertain and set in operation any adequate means of relief.

In former seasons, it has been usual to observe sporadic
cases of this disease for several weeks before the commencement of the epidemic. This was remarkably verified in
the late season; and such cases deserve the more attention
as they furnish the best means of calculating the probability
of approaching pestilence. Accordingly, one case of a decidedly malignant character was observed in the month of
June; several took place in July; a still greater number in
August; and at the beginning of September, they had become so numerous as to ascertain the existence of the epi-

demic. Throughout September and October, the disease continued to prevail with more or less severity according to the fluctuating states of the weather ; but towards the close of the latter month, the coldness of the season had evidently checked its progress ; and at the beginning of November, the city was nearly restored to usual health.

During the early period of the epidemic, nearly all the cases took place on the eastern side of the city, in Front, Water and Pearl streets, and principally below Burling-slip. They afterwards became more generally diffused. About the 20th of September, they began to prevail near the North River.* On the whole, the low grounds on the margin of the two rivers certainly produced a chief part of the cases. The number of deaths of the disease in the city, amounted to about 200; those at Bellevue Hospital to 52 ; and those at the Marine Hospital, sent from the city, to 28. The number of cases of malignant fever reported to the Board of Health amounted to about 600. It is proper, likewise, in estimating the extent of the epidemic, to notice an unascertained number, probably about 40, who after their flight from the city, died in various parts of the country.

The source of this disease forms a most interesting subject of inquiry ; on the success of which must depend all rational and adequate means of preventing and eradicating the evil. After a long and careful investigation of the subject, I cannot hesitate to conclude, that *a pernicious exhalation or*

---

* *A similar extension of the disease, in the epidemic of 1803, was ascribed by many to the removal of shipping from the East to the North river. As no such removal to that part of the city took place in the late season, it is necessary to explain the fact in some other way. This becomes very easy, when it is recollected that the made ground on the North river is much less extensive, and the materials composing it much less foul and corrupt, than that on the East river. The miasmata come to maturity on the one side two or three weeks sooner than on the other.*

vapour floating in the atmosphere, is the primary and essential cause of this disease. In order to produce this vapour, it is necessary that there should be a concurrence of heat, moisture, and a quantity of decaying animal and vegetable matter. It is therefore exhaled by heat from low and moist grounds, overspread with the corrupting offals of animal and vegetable substances, from such substances collected in large masses, or from any place where the process of putrefaction is going on to considerable extent. This exhalation likewise abounds more in some situations than in others. It is more frequently and copiously produced, and more highly concentrated, in warm and tropical countries than in high latitudes and frozen regions. It prevails and exerts its pernicious influence peculiarly in certain climates, seasons, and local situations. It is generated more in summer and operates more powerfully in autumn than in the other seasons of the year ; and it is uniformly more frequent and virulent in sea-port towns, in situations along sea-coasts, in plains, and near rivers, lakes, marshes and swamps, or wherever stagnant waters are found, than in the interior, high and mountainous districts of the country. It is undoubtedly one of the most universal causes of disease in nature. However diversified in quantity or virulence by local circumstances, or by varieties of climate, season or the condition of society, its effects in one degree or another are nearly co-extensive with the habitable parts of the globe.

While the noxious exhalation just described, when existing in a high degree of virulence, is considered as forming the primary and essential cause of our disease; it is proper, in order to be well understood, to notice the operation of certain *secondary* or *exciting causes.* These are exposure to heat, fatigue, cold, intemperance, fear, anxiety, &c. some of which are, in general, immediately instrumental in bringing on the disease in persons predisposed to it by the agency of the atmospheric poison. The noxiousness of this poison, by avoiding exciting causes, may often be long borne without falling into illness ; and hence the operation of exciting causes in suddenly producing the disease is often so striking as to lead many entirely to over-look the effect of the principal agent.

The sources of pernicious exhalation in this city are un-happily very numerous and difficult to correct. Some of them are evils of such magnitude and extent, that it re-quires resolution to consider them, and not to relinquish, in despair, the work of reformation. The mode of con-structing our wharves and slips would almost induce the belief that they had been designed for repositories of filth and nurseries of disease. The *made ground* on the East river is pregnant with almost annual pestilence ; it is now become enormously extensive ; it was originally composed of the most corrupt materials ; from its relation to the river, and the condition of the wharves and slips, it must constantly remain moist ; from its surface being nearly level, it receives and retains the collected filth washed down from the higher grounds ; and besides all this, the offensive and putrid matter, which a crowded population must necessarily deposit, and which already underlays a great proportion of this part of the city, incessantly aug-ments the mass of corruption. Can it possibly excite surprize, that the scorching heat of summer, operating on the complicated pollution of this ground, formed of an ag-gregate of nuisances, and still the receptacle of numberless others, should exhale poison and death into the atmosphere which stagnates over its surface?

As the materials of putrefaction and the degrees of heat, in a large city, greatly exceed what is found in the adja-cent country ; so the diseases arising under such circum-stances must be proportionably more malignant. The pes-tilential fevers of our city differ only in grade from the bilious and remittent fevers of the country. They prevail in the same climates ; they come on at the same season of the year; they are chiefly disposed to attack persons of the same constitution; they commit their ravages on the same organs of the body, and produce symptoms differing only in degree; and they decline and disappear at the same season and under the same circumstances. In the city we often see in the same family and under equal circumstances of exposure, the malignant forms of pestilence and the mild forms of remittent fever; and in the country, while the great mass of cases are usually mild, we occasionally meet with some which exhibit the violent attack, the intense malignity and the rapid dissolution, which more frequently mark the pestilential fevers of the city.

Besides the points of analogy just mentioned, there is another equally or perhaps more remarkable. The remittent fever of the country, and the malignant fevers (denominated *yellow*) of our cities, have a similar irregularity which generally characterizes them, and leads strongly to the inference of the similarity of their origin. In the districts of the country where remittent fevers prevail, and in the cities which produce malignant fevers, we find these diseases, in seasons apparently similar, and even in the same season, often exhibiting a singular local unsteadiness in their appearance, extent and violence. In the operation of the causes which produce them, there is something remarkably contingent and desultory. Remittent fevers will prevail sometimes in one district of a low country and sometimes in another; while the whole extent of these different districts seems to be equally liable to the disease, and no adequate cause can be assigned for the visitation of the one, and the escape of the other. In like manner, some of our cities are invaded by pestilence, in unfavorable seasons; while others, apparently just as liable to be invaded, escape.

For these reasons, as well as many others which my limits will not allow me to state, I conclude that our late epidemic, and all the preceding similar ones, have been of domestic

G

origin, and, of course, nearly related to the remittent bilious fevers of the country.

From this simple and consistent view of the subject, the
attention of some has been unfortunately drawn aside by the
mistaken opinions of the *importation of the disease from a-
broad*, and *the propagation of it by contagion*.

I. As the question of contagion, in this disease, is important
and fundamental, and as the affirmative has been asserted
with much confidence, it becomes necessary to consider this
point with great attention.

But, before proceeding to offer reasons in detail against
the contagiousness of yellow fever, it is proper to premise
some general observations on the subject.

A contagious disease is distinguished from all others by
the property of generating or secreting a matter, which, applied by contact, or inhaled with the air by near approach to
the sick or to inanimate substances charged with their effluvia,
successively reproduces the same disease. As this contagious matter is secreted by a morbid action of vessels, or a
peculiar process of the disease, forming a specific and essential part of its character, it must always be generated when
such disease exists ; and being generated, and then duly applied or inhaled, its action is altogether independent of external circumstances, such as the state of the air, &c. and
must always take effect, unless there be something in the
condition of persons exposed to it, which renders them un-
susceptible of the impression. This unsusceptibility, depending upon peculiar and unusual circumstances, (except
in the diseases which attack the same person but once,) must
of course be extremely rare. The small pox affords an example of this operation of contagion. If forty persons, who
have never undergone small pox, be closely exposed to the
effluvia of a number of patients lying ill of that disease in
the ward of a small pox hospital, thirty-nine certainly, and
probably the whole number, will be infected. This is an example of a contagious distemper. The contagious matter

is the constant and universal product of the disease; and when produced, it generally reproduces itself in such as receive it; provided they have not been (in the case of small pox) previously subjected to its action. The principle of unsusceptibility cannot reside in the surrounding air, but is to be sought for in the body that resists the contagion. There are no facts to prove that pure atmospheric air is a neutralizer or destroyer of contagion; every day presents instances of the reverse; and when diffused through an extensive space, air renders it harmless, not by immediately decomposing, but by diluting and dissipating it. On the other hand, none of the truly contagious diseases derive any additional force from impure air; for the greater contagiousness of confined air in cases of this sort, arises merely from the concentration of a greater quantity of contagious matter within a small space. The application of these principles to the subject in question will presently be seen.

It is proper likewise to premise, that the attack of many persons in the same neighbourhood, or even of whole families, by a reigning disease, affords no proof of contagion* ; for the intermittent and remittent bilious fevers of the country, which undoubtedly are not propagated by contagion, often attack families and neighborhoods so generally as scarcely to leave healthy persons in sufficient number to attend the sick.

* *In the course of the autumn, about five years ago, ninety-eight out of a hundred of the labourers employed at the* Onondaga Salt-Works, *in this State, were attacked with bilious fever. The two who escaped, probably owed their exemption to extensive ulcers with which they happened, at that time, to be affected. That situation is unusually sickly in the summer and autumn; and a large proportion of the cases of fever which occur there, become malignant and fatal. By the death of several persons, within a few years, who held the office of Superintendant of the Works, and who fell victims to this malignant fever in close succession, that station is now justly regarded by the people of the neighbouring districts, as extremely hazardous.*

The want of due discrimination between the effects of an *impure atmosphere* and of *contagion*, is one of the most lamentable deficiencies in the history of diseases.*

The agency of contagion in the propagation of our malignant disease is rejected for the following reasons.

1. No relation is observed between the source of the pretended contagion, and the spreading of the disease to individuals or families ; nor was there ever any foundation to attempt progressively to trace the propagation of it to any number of persons, from the first case, or from any single point of infection. If the first ten or twenty cases, which occur in any season, be strictly scrutinized, most of them are found, in their origin, to be distinct and independent of one another. Instead of pervading families, or creeping slowly from one neighbourhood to another, in the track of infection, as is invariably the case with contagious distempers, this disease is found scattered at distant and unconnected points, and cases start up singly in situations where contagion could neither be traced nor suspected.† The pro-

---

* *Some epidemic diseases, such as small pox, &c. are considered, by universal consent, as contagious ; others, such as bilious remittent fevers, &c. are considered as non-contagious. It becomes, therefore, extremely interesting to ascertain the criteria by which this discrimination among epidemic distempers may be clearly and promptly made. The want of precision on this point has produced much collision of opinion and much absurdity of conduct among physicians and others. The most obvious criterion, and that which is most generally recognized by the common sense of mankind, is the effect of personal intercourse between the sick and the well. Where a disease is truly contagious, this intercourse cannot fail to disclose the danger, which was long ago correctly stated in poetical language :*

    " Quo propior quisque est, servitque fidelius ægro,
    " In partem lethi citius venit."

                         Ovid. Metamorph. lib. 7.

† *Not only the dispersion of the cases is adverse to the doctrine of contagion ; but the appearance of them in groups in some*

portion of single cases in the midst of families is always great ; and the instances of any large proportion of families being attacked were comparatively very rare in our late epidemic. It appears from the records of this epidemic, that there were thirty-one streets of the city, most of which continued to be crowded with inhabitants, in which only a single case in each occurred ; and in the mass of six hundred cases, reported to the Board of Health, there were only thirty-five houses in which more than a single case was found. If the number of deaths should be supposed to afford better ground of calculation, it will be found that there were forty streets, and those generally crowded throughout the season, in which only one death in each took place ; not more than three died in one house, of which there were only two instances ; and, during the whole epidemic, there were only twelve instances of two persons dying in one house.* The great mass of persons attacked with the disease, consisted of such as never had approached the sick, or any other assignable source of contagion ; and, on the contrary, as will presently appear, great numbers were exposed to close intercourse with the sick, without injury.

instances is altogether as much so. Many of the most judicious of our citizens were convinced of the origination of the disease from domestic filth in the year 1798, by the following occurrence. Between twenty and thirty persons, at the commencement of that destructive epidemic, in a small neighbourhood at the lower end of John-street, were suddenly seized with the disease in one night, in consequence of a blast of putrid exhalations from the sewer of Burling-slip. The persons attacked were only such as lived directly to the leeward of this blast from the sewer ; while others, close in the vicinity, but not exposed to this current, entirely escaped.

* From these reports to the Board of Health, it results that upwards of five hundred, out of six hundred cases of malignant fever which occurred, were single in the respective families ; and that more than three-fourths of the deaths which took place in the city, were likewise single in the respective families in which they occurred.

In order to explain this scattered, remote and unconnected occurrence of cases, the advocates of contagion are obliged to resort to the extravagant supposition of the contagion
being diffused through an extensive range of atmosphere,
or, to use their own singular phrase, of an *inoculation of
the atmosphere* by the effluvia of the sick, or of the infected
cloathing or bedding which were supposed originally to have
introduced the contagion. It is scarcely necessary to observe, that this is a new and unheard of doctrine, utterly
unknown and repugnant to all the principles and laws of the
communication of contagion, which have been sanctioned by
the experience of ages, and entirely subversive of all the
hopes the contagionists themselves can repose on a separation of the sick from the well, or on the most rigid regulations of quarantine. This doctrine is likewise inconsistent
with itself. If contagion from a single source can extend
itself so far, what would become of the inhabitants of the
city generally, when, in the progress of the epidemic, cases
are so immensely multiplied, and the disease so extremely
diffused? If this contagion can exercise such a destructive
activity at a distance, after being so much diluted in the air,
what must be the effect of approaching near to the source?
If a contagion really existed, capable of retaining its virulence, after such extensive diffusion in the atmosphere, it
would bid defiance to all the barriers of quarantine, be inco-
ercible by human means, and finally would depopulate the
world. Another inconsistency is equally glaring. If this
effluvium from a sick body, or from foul cloathing and bedding, can be supposed to vitiate the air to such a distance
around, it must, after such extensive diffusion, become light
and fugitive, and liable to be blown away by the first breeze.
But, how does it happen that this same space of air, after
the inhabitants are fled, the sick removed, and houses shut
up, continues, till a change of season, to be permanently
noxious? Nothing can account for this local, stationary and
inexhaustible poison, but the exhalations from the masses of

filth and pollution overspreading a large area of ground, forming a vast hot-bed of putrefaction, incessantly teeming with miasmata, and thereby, in despite of currents of air, loading with the seeds of disease every successive portion of atmosphere that sweeps or stagnates over the pestilential surface.

2. The pretended contagion is admitted to produce no effect in our climate, except in particular situations, and at a particular season of the year, when an impure and noxious atmosphere, which ought to be considered as a sufficient cause, is acknowledged to exist. But to consider a disease as contagious, which at the same time exhibits no appearance of that quality but in certain climates, in such climates only in certain places, at such places only at certain seasons, and even at such seasons only after a particular degree of heat and moisture, is undoubtedly to lose sight of all the established properties and laws of contagion.

3. It is admitted that the disease does not spread when the sick are removed from the impure air in which it was contracted. By breathing this impure air, without exposure to the effluvia of the sick, persons are every day attacked ; while, on the contrary, without breathing it, however exposed to such effluvia, no person is attacked. The conclusion, therefore, is irresistible, that the impure air is the cause.

4. No communication of the disease was ever observed in yellow fever hospitals, situated at a small distance from the cities to which they belong. No exception to this has ever occurred in any of the numerous seasons of this pestilence at our hospital at Bellevue, the Marine Hospital at Staten-Island,* that of Philadelphia, or any other in the United

* *The two pretended cases of contagion at the Marine Hospital on Staten Island, one in the year* 1799 *and the other in* 1800, *were evidently fevers produced by the poison of typhus, modified by the season. Nature is too simple and uniform in her operations to constitute a disease contagious, and yet only so once in a thousand instances.*

States; provided the malignant air of the city had been avoided. The force of this fact seems never to have been duly considered or appreciated. The numerous retinue of medical attendants, nurses, washerwomen, servants, &c. which belong to a hospital, must be known to every body. How greatly they are all exposed to contagion, if it could be supposed to exist in this case, is equally known. The most malignant degrees of the disease are constantly found in these institutions. The exposure of physicians and their assistants is well understood. The duty of the nurses leads to an incessant and unreserved intercourse with the sick. They pass the greater part of their time, and sleep in the apartments of the sick, the dying and the dead.* In lifting, undressing, dressing, administering remedies, and many other modes of assistance, they are very often in actual contact, and commonly within a small distance of the patients. They receive and carry away all excrementitious discharges. Several persons are employed in washing the foul clothes and bedding of the sick and the dead. Not only all these have invariably escaped the disease, but likewise all the persons occupied in the removal of the sick from the city to the hospital, who in this service went without reserve into the most pestilential quarters of the town, entered the most filthy apartments, and lifted the sick into their carriages dressed in their foulest clothes, and sinking under the worst degrees of the disease.†

* *The nurses at Bellevue Hospital became so entirely free from all apprehensions of the contagiousness of this disease, that they often slept on the same bed with the sick; and it happened more than once, in the course of the season, that a nurse, overcome with fatigue and want of sleep, threw herself in the night, for a little repose, on the bed of a dying patient, and remained there asleep till the patient was dead, and it became necessary to remove the corpse.*

† *In order to account for the escape of these persons, which is indeed wonderful, it is proper to state that they all resided during the season at the Alms-House, an elevated*

In order to account for these facts, the advocates of contagion contend that its activity is confined to *impure air*, and
that by this alone it can be *conducted* to the objects of its attack. Our hospital at Bellevue, however, is not so constructed as to allow the supposition of great purity of the air ; and
indeed the state of the land-air in the months of August,
September and October, cannot be considered as pure, in
any part of our country. But admitting the highest possible purity of air in these hospitals, the operation of contagion,
if it existed there, could not by such means be avoided.
When the naked hands of physicians and nurses are in contact with the skin of the patient, scorched with febrile heat,
or bedewed with the matter of perspiration, how can pure
air be interposed to arrest the passage of contagion ? When
they inhale, as they often do, the breath and effluvia of the
sick, no man can doubt that such air is sufficiently impure to
be the *conductor* of contagion, if it really existed. In all
contagious diseases, contact and immediate inhalation of the
effluvia and breath of the sick, are supposed to constitute
the greatest possible exposure ; and in such cases, it is plain,
the interposition of air, pure or impure, must be equally un-
availing to arrest the evil. Yet in these hospitals, persons
not only escape this danger, but none was ever known to be
infected by it.‡

5. The extinction of the disease by cold weather, is an
insuperable objection to the doctrine of its propagation by

*and healthy part of the city, and consequently were only
for a short period, at any one time, immersed in the noxious
atmosphere.*

‡ *In the epidemic of the year* 1798, *seven persons died of
Yellow Fever in our Alms-House. It was ascertained that
they had taken the disease in consequence of going out and
breathing the atmospheric poison diffused through the more
contaminated districts of the city. Although the house then
contained about* 800 *persons, no communication of contagion
took place.*

H

contagion. That the disease in reality depends upon an atmospheric poison, appears from the fact, that all the means which operate to arrest and destroy it, such as cold, heavy rains and high winds, are merely atmospheric agents. The healthy temperature of the human body is the same in all climates and seasons; and febrile heat is not less in winter than summer. Consequently, the morbid process by which the matter of contagion is generated, is under no controul from atmospheric temperature. Hot climates and seasons are universally held to be unfavorable to the spreading of contagion. The reason is obvious. In warm weather, the doors and windows of the apartments of the sick are kept open, and ventilation is carried to the highest degree. At this season, the effluvia of the body, whether in health or disease, are sooner dissipated, and, of course, can less readily adhere to clothing, bedding, walls, furniture, &c. so as to be retained, and become noxious. In conformity to this, typhus, which is propagated by a poison produced in the clothing, bedding, furniture, &c. of persons living in filthy and crowded apartments, generally prevails and spreads much more in winter, when such apartments are deprived of ventilation. On the contrary, yellow fever, arising from a deleterious principle floating in the atmosphere, and produced by the operation of solar heat upon vegetable and animal filth, ceases to prevail soon after this heat is reduced so low that it can no longer exhale a sufficient quantity of the miasmata of putrefaction. But if this disease depended upon contagion, instead of disappearing at the accession of cold weather, when houses are more closely shut up, it would be then more certainly communicated, and more widely destructive.

6. Yellow fever does not prevail in countries, where the heat is not sufficient to exhale the miasmata of putrefaction, in the requisite quantity and virulence. We hear nothing of this disease in Great Britain, Ireland, or France; though it is well known that persons ill of it, and shipping

in which it has recently prevailed, very frequently arrive in their ports. The boarding houses in the sea-port towns of these countries, in which seamen arriving from the West-Indies are generally lodged, are known to be often extremely filthy and filled with impure air ; as appears from the prevalence and ravages of typhus ; yet this impure air in those countries cannot *conduct* the contagion of yellow fever.

7. Many persons, who had contracted the disease in New-York, died of it at Boston, Albany and other cities at a distance ; many likewise at Greenwich, Brooklyn, and other villages in the neighbourhood. In no instance did these victims of the epidemic communicate contagion. In all these places, the air at that season must have been very *impure*; at Albany and Brooklyn violent remittent fevers were at the same time extremely prevalent; and yet this impurity of the air did not serve as a *conductor* of contagion.

8. Among the early cases of this disease, in the late season, which were, as usual, most virulent, very striking examples of its non-contagiousness were displayed in some of the most crowded quarters of the city. In the beginning of September, a considerable number of sick, who had taken the disease on the eastern side of the city, were removed to the western side ; where they died with the most pestilential symptoms. In a house in Cedar-street, where two patients expired under the worst symptoms of this description, the *beds of the deceased, in a very few hours after their death, were occupied by the survivors

* *It is proper to observe that, since the first publication of this letter, a contradiction of the statement concerning the beds has been received from one person, and a confirmation of it from another. That particular circumstance is, however, immaterial ; as it is admitted on all hands that no contagion arose from either of these malignant cases.*

of the family. Yet in none of these numerous instances was any contagion communicated.

9. The universal exemption of the physicians of New-York, amounting at least to 50 or 60 persons, from the late disease, is also irreconcilable with the doctrine of its contagiousness. I have not heard of any physician in Philadelphia, New-Haven, Providence or Norfolk, suffering illness from their late epidemics. It is known that physicians neither use nor possess antidotes. Their exposure to the breath, effluvia and contact of the sick, was almost incessant from morning till night. They employed no precaution of dress or covering, no fumigation, no means of destroying neutralizing or obviating, in any manner, the effluvia of their patients. The dissection of bodies dead of Yellow Fever, if contagion had existed, would also have formed another source of danger. Many of the physicians of this city were frequently engaged in this mode of investigating the disease, and minutely examined bodies in a very advanced state of putridity. The more happy escape of physicians in the late than in former epidemics, is to be attributed (under the protection of Divine Providence) to their having secured a residence in the higher and safer parts of the town, and to the comparative infrequency of their visits to the districts of envenomed atmosphere ; owing to the early desertion of these districts by the chief part of the inhabitants. It is understood, at the same time, that our physicians, in their confidence of the non-contagiousness of the disease, generally passed more time in the apartments of the sick, and were in the habit of making a more deliberate and minute examination of the cases which fell under their care, than in preceding epidemics.*

* *The exemption of the nurses from disease, who attended the sick in the city, was also very remarkable. Upwards of sixty persons were employed, by the Board of Health, to perform this duty. Only four of these died ; two others only were*

10. The failure of every attempt to arrest the progress of the disease, by the separation of the sick from the well, is also incompatible with the doctrine of contagion. Besides the numerous ineffectual attempts in this city, the utmost endeavours were used, with the same result, by the Board of Health of Philadelphia, whose members had been purposely selected for this object, from those who embraced the opinion of the importation and contagiousness of the disease. It would be fortunate, indeed, for the purpose of arresting Yellow Fever, if its progress depended upon contagion. This appears from the example of the small pox, a disease whose contagion is more active, steady and permanent than any other in the world. By a system of quarantine, extremely simple and very little burthensome, this distemper is excluded, or, if introduced, immediately arrested and banished, in Boston and other cities of New-England, where its admission and circulation are prohibited by law.

11. The inconsistency and contradiction which constantly attend the application of the doctrine of contagion in this disease, make it altogether inadmissible. To explain one set of facts, it must infinitely transcend the contagiousness of small pox; to suit another, it must sink infinitely in the opposite direction. On some occasions, it is more subtle, penetrating and rapid than the electric fluid; on others, more sluggish and dormant than the grossest matter. Contrary to all other noxious substances, it is often more destructive at a distance, than near to its source; for at one time, it cannot reach a single individual among a great number surrounding the bed of the patient, and in frequent contact with his person, while at another, it must strike at the distance of several hundred feet.* THE

sick, and recovered. And it appears, upon inquiry, that such as died or were sick, had been stationed in the parts of the city where the atmosphere was known to be most highly charged with the miasmata of putrefaction.

* While it is admitted that contagion cannot operate in

NOXIOUSNESS OF THE MIASMATA OF PUTREFACTION, EX-
HALED BY HEAT AND FLOATING IN THE ATMOSPHERE,
EXPLAINS ALL THESE FACTS, AND RECONCILES ALL THESE
CONTRADICTIONS.

If it were possible to add any thing to the evidence of
these irresistiblœ facts, I might subjoin, that Yellow Fever
cannot be considered as a contagious disease ;—Because,
unlike all other contagious diseases, it has no specific character, no definite course or duration, and no appropriate,
essential or pathognomonic symptom ;—Because, the supposed contagion rarely operates singly, and in general depends upon the co-operation of exciting causes ;—and finally, Because, the miasmata which produce this disease are
more or less noxious as they are more or less concentrated,
a property which does not belong to the specific poisons of
small pox, syphilis, &c.

Under the conviction of these facts, I am compelled to
conclude that our malignant disease is the effect of a noxious exhalation floating in the atmosphere, and that it is
ABSOLUTELY AND UNIVERSALLY NON-CONTAGIOUS.

For the correctness of the facts on which this conclusion is
founded, I appeal to my fellow-practitioners and fellow-citizens, who have been witnesses of the disease. For the application of these facts in the deduction of principles and
opinions, I appeal to the judgment of physicians in every
quarter of the world, where Medicine is cultivated as a regular science. And, especially, I would offer this appeal

*Yellow Fever Hospitals, and while this inactivity of it is
ascribed to the absence of impure air; it is, at the same
time, gravely asserted by some that a person going on board of
a vessel, lying in a situation where the air is much more pure
than it can possibly be at a hospital, even though there exist
no sickness on board of such vessel, may still derive contagion from it, and experience all the active and malignant
operation of such contagion, notwithstanding this purity
of the surrounding atmosphere.*

to the liberal and enlightened physicians of Europe, who are sincerely devoted to the cause of truth and professional improvement, who, on this subject, have heretofore received much incorrect information, and who, as soon as they become convinced of the real state of the question, will, I am confident, exert the influence they so justly possess, in procuring from their respective Governments an abolition of the oppressive and useless restrictions of quarantine, which have been recently imposed on American commerce.

II. The second mistake concerning this malignant disease, which has been impressed on the minds of some of our citizens, is that of its *importation from abroad, and chiefly from the West-Indies.* This opinion is rejected for the following reasons :

1. The non-contagiousness of the disease must entirely destroy the belief of its introduction from abroad. It is impossible to conceive that it can be conveyed across the ocean, and propagated in the cities of the United States, unless it possess the power of successively re-producing itself by communication of contagion from one person to another.

2. If the alleged importation were possible in any case, it might happen at any season of the year. In this active sea-port, shipping from the West-Indies are very frequently arriving at all seasons ; and it is known that yellow fever may be found in those islands at any period of the year, when they are visited by strangers from the higher latitudes : yet the pretended importation is always confined to that period of the summer and autumn, when local and domestic causes, sufficient to produce the disease, are known to exist.

3. If yellow fever could be introduced from abroad, it is impossible to explain its non-appearance in our sea-ports for a long series of years, when no means were used to secure its exclusion. For more than fifty years preceding 1795, no importation of the disease into this city was suspected ; and it is indeed uncertain whether, before that year, the opinion

of its importation at any period of the eighteenth century, had attracted much attention. The advocates of importation generally assert, that periods of war in the W. Indies are most apt to occasion its introduction into this country. Yet we hear nothing of its being brought to this port during the war of 1756, or that of the American Revolution. In the former of these wars, the mortality attending the successful expeditions against Martinique, Guadaloupe and the Havanna, was almost incredible. Only a very small part of the victorious troops were alive three months after their conquests. Equally fatal were the malignant fevers of the West-Indies in the war of the American Revolution. Dr. Hunter* informs us, that of 5,000 troops who took possession of St. Lucie, scarcely a man of the original number remained at the end of one year; although the sword of the enemy had destroyed an inconsiderable amount. The mortality continued as great in the subsequent years. From the 1st of May 1780, to the 1st of May 1781, the number of dead was equal to the average strength of the garrison during the year. Of the troops sent from Jamaica upon the expedition against Fort St. Juan, scarcely a man ever returned. During this period, the intercourse between the West-Indies and this port, must have been extremely frequent. Doctor Blane† states, that in the course of the war of our Revolution, nearly 18,000 sick were landed at New-York from the British fleets; that 11 sail of the line arrived here early in September 1780, from the W. Indies; that 26 sail of the line arrived here at the same season in 1782, likewise from the W. Indies; and that from each of these fleets, a great number of sick, afflicted with malignant fevers, were sent to the hospitals at this place. It is also known that a similar fleet arrived here in the beginning of the autumn of the year 1781. During all this period, notwithstanding the ravages of yellow fever

* *Observations on the Diseases of the Army in Jamaica.*
† *Observations on the Diseases of Seamen.*

in the West-Indies, and the conveyance of so many sick to this port, we hear nothing of the importation of the disease. And yet, at that time, no quarantine-regulations existed.

The contingencies by which yellow fever might have been imported, through the medium of commercial shipping or of naval and military expeditions, if such importation were possible, must very often have occurred in a sea-port like this, where such extensive communication has been so long maintained with the West-Indies. A more frequent introduction of the disease, therefore, according to the doctrine of importation, as now held, must have been inevitable. But as this did not take place for such a length of time, and under circumstances so likely to produce it, we are warranted in the conclusion that importation is impossible.

On the contrary, as the history of pestilential epidemics in all ages and countries demonstrates that they are subject to frequent revolutions, as to the periods and places of their prevalence, the variety of their symptoms and the degrees of their malignity ; it is much more easy to account for changes in such diseases, as they locally or periodically occur, than for any great diversity or fluctuation in the circumstances or contingencies, which determine their importation from abroad.

4. No importation of this disease, so as to become epidemic, was ever known in any port of Great Britain, Ireland or France. The vast amount of shipping, as was observed before, which arrive at those ports from the West-Indies, is well known ; and, that they often arrive in a very sickly condition, is equally known. The filth and impure air of those ports are admitted on all hands, and the effects of them are experienced in the destructive fevers of a different description which frequently prevail ; and yet, for want of the atmospheric heat and other local circumstances requisite in the generation of yellow fever, they are happily strangers to its epidemic prevalence.

5. The appearance of yellow fever in many of the interior

I

parts of the country, inaccessible to foreign contagion, con-firms the opinion of its domestic origin, while it entirely in-validates that of its importation. There is not a State in the Union, which has not afforded evidence of the production of the disease, in situations where importation was impracticable. In the course of the late season, a malignant fever, in all essential points the same as our yellow fever, prevailed in many parts of this State, and caused more mortality, in pro-portion to the population of the district, than took place in this city. There can be no reasonable doubt, that the disease called the *Lake Fever*, in the interior of this State, possesses all the essential attributes of the yellow fever.

6. A comparison of the summer and autumn of the year 1804, with the corresponding seasons in 1805, will go far to shew the dependence of our malignant epidemics on the con-dition of the atmosphere, and, of course, to overthrow the doctrine of importation. The summer of 1804 was mild and cool, beyond former example, on all the Atlantic coast of the United States, lying to the northward of the Caro-linas. In South-Carolina and Georgia, the heat was unusu-ally great. All the Atlantic cities north of the Carolinas, without exception, entirely escaped the epidemic: whereas at Charleston and in some parts of Georgia, it prevailed with great mortality. On the contrary, the late summer was re-markable for the duration as well as the intensity of heat, along the whole of our coast. And the consequence was, not only that nearly all the Atlantic cities were visited with pestilence, but, what was still more surprising, that in seve-ral of them it made its appearance within forty-eight hours, or nearly, of the same time ; an occurrence which cannot be explained on the contingency of importation, and is only to be satisfactorily accounted for from the state of the atmos-phere.

7. The occurrence of similar diseases in other parts of the world, under similar circumstances, where contagion intro-ced from abroad cannot possibly be suspected, is also ad-verse to the doctrine of importation. In making the circuit

of the globe, on the parallels of latitude nearly or exactly corresponding with ours, we pass over countries which, from the earliest records of history, have been frequently visited with the ravages of this scourge. Spain and Italy afford striking examples. The city of Rome, in particular, though its elevated situation is generally salubrious, is annoyed by a marshy spot at the feet of two of its hills, along the margin of the Tiber, which has been sickly and pestilential from the origin of the city. While the streets on the hills, like Broadway and other high grounds in this city, enjoy a salubrious air, the spot of marsh just mentioned, together with a small extent of *made-ground*, (for the madness of *made-ground* has existed at Rome as well as at New-York*), corresponding with our marshy districts and vastly more extended space of made-ground, along the margin of the East-River, has produced, from time immemorial, malignant and mortal epidemics. And the medical historian of these facts, (the celebrated Baglivi) expresses his astonishment that so small a distance, as that intervening between the elevated and depressed portions of ground, should make such a difference in the qualities of the air. As the Tiber is not navigable for sea-vessels, the importation of their pestilential epidemics at Rome was never suggested.

8. The inefficacy of all the various modifications of quarantine hitherto devised in this country, confirms our disbelief of importation. In this port, as well as in Philadelphia,

---

**Proofs of this might be adduced from Lancisi and other medical writers of Rome. The following lines are sufficient to establish the fact :*

> Hoc, ubi nunc fora sunt, udæ tenuere paludes;
> Amne redundatis fossa madebat aquis.
> Curtius illo lacus, siccas qui sustinet aras,
> Nunc solida est tellus, sed lacus ante fuit.
> Quà Velabra solent in Circum ducere pompas,
> Nil præter salices cassaque canna fuit.

Ovid. Fast. Lib. VI.

a rigid system of quarantine has been in operation for many years; and there is no doubt of its having been vigilantly and faithfully executed. Indeed, the experience of quarantine in the United States speaks little in its favor; for though, during the last ten years, it has been scrupulously enforced in several ports, we have heard ten times more of imported contagion and of its ravages, at these very ports, during that short period, than for an hundred years before, when no quarantine was in existence.

9. The entire want of all proof, and even of the least probability of the introduction from abroad of the germ of our late epidemic, gives the last blow to the doctrine of importation. The facts on this subject have been so clearly and minutely detailed by the Health Officer, that it would be superfluous to repeat them here.

The source of mistake, on the subject of importation, consists in not distinguishing *a febrile poison generated by heat and filth in a vessel*, from *contagion taken up in a foreign port, and successively communicated from one person to another*. The construction of vessels disposes them to the collection and retention of filth, and renders cleansing and ventilation extremely difficult. The quality of cargoes and provisions, the inattention of seamen to cleanliness, the crowded manner in which they often live, the unsuspected and inaccessible situations in which corrupting substances may lie concealed, render shipping, independently of the hazards of the element on which they move, the most dangerous of all human habitations. It is no wonder, therefore, that they should become unhealthy, when they pass into warm latitudes, or lie in our harbour in the hot season. In no situation is a malignant fever more apt to originate than in a ship. A vessel that never left our port, or that has remained in it for years, may become foul and thereby generate and emit a deadly exhalation. Whether malignant fever arise from filth ashore or on shipboard, the principles and process, by which the evil is produced, are still the same. On what ground can a disease be said to be *imported*, which has no other relation to a foreign country, than that of being generated in a vessel which has lately visited that country ? The foreign country, the outward and homeward voyage, are circumstances of no moment in determining the origin and character of the disease; to account for this, we must consider the filth, the moisture and heat, which, concurring to a certain degree, are destructive to man at all times, in all situations and under every condition. And a fever originating under such circumstances, can no more be pronounced *imported*, than a fracture of a limb happening at sea can be called an *imported fracture*.

It has been supposed by some, who regard only one aspect of the subject, that the doctrine of importation alone can explain the more frequent recurrence of malignant epidemics for the last ten years. But the difficulty still returns with unabated force; and it remains to explain, why importation has become so much more frequent and easy of late than formerly. If it be thought impracticable to throw light on that peculiar constitution of the air, which determines the prevalence of yellow fever at one time more than another; it is equally impracticable to ascertain the qualities of the air which produce malignant distempers of the throat, the dysentery, and other mortal epidemics, (which are undoubtedly of domestic origin) for a season, or for a term of years, and then allow them to disappear.

It has been said, that the belief of the yellow fever originating in this country, would be destructive to its commerce and prosperity. But if the appeal must be made to interest rather than truth, let us contrast the effects of the two opinions, as they influence our intercourse with foreign nations. By truly describing the disease, and exhibiting the proofs of its local origin and non-contagiousness, we convince foreign nations that it is a misfortune limited to ourselves, that it cannot endanger their safety, and that it only claims their sympathy and regrets. By asserting the importation and contagiousness of it, the evil immediately swells to an indefinite and incalculable extent, and we alarm all nations with the fear of its being, in turn, exported to them. After the experience already gained, neither they nor we can cherish any rational hope of hereafter excluding it, by regulations of quarantine. Our intercourse with the West-Indies, and with all other tropical countries, will be daily extended, and if importation were possible, the chances of it will be every year progressively multiplied. On the ground of importation, unless trade be totally forsaken, our situation is hopeless.

In rejecting the doctrine of importation, the benefits of quarantine are by no means intended to be undervalued. The generation of pestilential disease in foul vessels is undeniable ; they are certainly a very frequent source of sickness ; and all persons concerned in shipping are interested in a careful examination of them. There ought to be some mode of ascertaining whether a vessel may be safely approached by people in business, or whether she may be likely to diffuse pestilential vapours among all who come within their reach. Quarantine is also one of the most humane regulations in favor of seamen, who are confessedly a very useful and necessary class of the community. It interposes between them and the carelessness or cruelty of their commander, and makes it his interest to preserve their lives and health. And while it might be organized so as to answer all these purposes efficaciously, it might also be properly stripped of its useless and burthensome appendages.

If the facts and reasonings, which I have adduced to prove the non-contagiousness and non-importation of yellow fever, be well founded, it results that our epidemics are local, domestic, and as incapable of exportation to foreign nations, as the bilious fever of the country. It is to be lamented that the reverse of this opinion has made so deep an impression in Europe ; and that the Governments of that quarter of the world have suffered themselves so lightly and hastily to embrace doctrines and legislate on principles contradicted by all former experience. It is now more than 300 years since they became acquainted with America. And although the first discoverers of the new world, as well as most succeeding adventurers, have largely shared the effects of the baneful climate of the West-Indies ; it is only of late that apprehensions have been entertained of importing into Europe the malignant fevers of those islands. The shattered remains of fleets and armies had often returned home to Great-Britain and France, in the most sickly state, after encountering all the horrors of yellow fever, without once communicating that disease. But what transmutation can yellow fever undergo in the United States, which renders it exportable to Europe from us, but not directly from the West-Indies ?

It affords some apology indeed for Europe, that the information concerning this subject, upon which they have acted, was derived from our own country. The acts of our State Legislatures, the proceedings of our Municipal Bodies and Boards of Health, the proclamations of our Magistrates, and a variety of other public documents, have all a tendency to impress the same opinion. We have held up to foreign nations, an indigenous and local disease, growing up from the infelicities of particular situations, or from neglects of police, and entirely incommunicable from one person to another, as highly contagious, capable of exportation to distant countries, and consequently alarming to the safety of the whole commercial and civilized world. We cannot transplant the disease from this city to the neighbouring villages of Greenwich, Brooklyn, or Newark ; and yet it is believed we can convey it 3000 miles across the pure air of the Atlantic. Whole hospitals of patients, labouring under the most malignant forms of the disease, with all the foul apparel, bedding, &c. polluted with the excrementitious discharges and other filth of the sick, the dying and the dead, cannot emit an atom of contagion ; and yet we pretend to dread the infectiousness of a sailor's jacket or handkerchief, or even of the cordage and timbers of a vessel. Under the influence of this phantom of contagion, we have instructed the Europeans to enact laws and regulations, sanctioned by the highest penalties, which retard and oppress our commerce, and subject our shipping in their ports to the most grievous detention. To crown the whole of this injury and humiliation, we have instigated them to place the people of the United States, by late extensions of quarantine, on the same footing with the degraded and detestable inhabitants of Barbary, Egypt, Syria, the Archipelago, Constantinople and other parts of the Turkish dominions. And all this has been done, in defiance of clear and luminous facts, and in the face of long, reiterated and ample experience.

By discarding the bugbear of contagion, the origin and nature of Yellow Fever will be more truly ascertained; the means of personal safety more generally understood; and the measures necessary to improve the salubrity of the city more vigorously pursued. The public will no longer witness that desertion and misery of the sick, which have too often disgraced society, in every epidemic. The bosom of humanity will no longer be wrung with the sufferings of our fellow-creatures, driven, while under the pressure of this calamity, from every place of shelter, deprived of comfort, and abandoned to their fate, from the false impression of danger in affording them assistance. By telling the community the truth, we shall lessen apprehension and distress, we shall disarm the evil of half its power, and restore the ties of kindred, and of nature.*

---

* *The learned* DR. HUNTER, *one of the members of the* NATIONAL BOARD OF HEALTH *of Great Britain, offers the following argument in support of his opinion of the non-contagiousness of Yellow Fever.* " *The strongest proofs of this, in my opinion, were to be met with in private families, where the son, the brother, or the husband, labouring under the worst fevers, were nursed with unremitting assiduity by the mother, the sister, or the wife, who never left the sick either by day or by night, yet without being infected. That such near relations should take upon them the*

It is surely time to investigate this subject with the deep-
est attention, and to adopt some adequate system of relief.
The warning voice of history and experience loudly calls us
to make every exertion to deliver our city from nuisances,
which threaten to entail the miseries of an annual succession
of malignant epidemics. WE LIVE IN THE LATITUDE OF
PESTILENCE, AND OUR CLIMATE NOW PERHAPS IS ONLY
BEGINNING TO DISPLAY ITS TENDENCY TO PRODUCE THIS
TERRIBLE SCOURGE.† The impurities, which time and
a police, rather moulded in conformity to the usages
of more northern countries than to the exigencies of
our own, have been long accumulating, are now annu-

*office of a nurse, is matter of the highest commendation in
a country, the diseases of which require to be watched with
greater care and attention than can be expected from a servant. They are under no fears of the fever being infectious, and I never saw any reason to believe it to be so, either
in private families, or in the military hospitals." That
Dr. Hunter came to this decision, after a full and mature
consideration of the importance of the subject, will appear
from the following remarks : " There is hardly any part
of the history of a disease, which it is of more consequence
to ascertain with accuracy, than its being of an infectious
nature, or not. Upon this depends the propriety of the
steps that should be taken, either to prevent it, or to root it
out. It is productive of great mischief to consider a disease as infectious, that really is not so ; it exposes such as
labour under it to evils and inconveniencies, which greatly
aggravate their sufferings, and often deprive them of the
necessary assistance. They are neglected, if not shunned ;
and at the time they require the greatest care and attention,
they have the least."*
Observ. on the Diseases of the Army in Jamaica, page 177 & 178.

† To convince the reader of this, it is only necessary
to remind him how near the cities of Philadelphia and
New-York lie to the parallels on which Rome and Constantinople are situated. It is scarcely requisite to observe,
that the ravages of pestilence in these ancient cities have
far exceeded any thing which has occurred elsewhere, unless
those of Grand Cairo should be supposed to equal them.

K

ally exposed to the heats of a burning summer, and send forth exhalations of the highest virulence. The examples of similar calamities in many parts of the old continent, ought long since to have taught us lessons of wisdom. In the city of Rome, time and fatal experience pointed out the necessity of erecting extensive and costly public works, in order to deliver the inhabitants from the horrors of pestilence ; and the air of that City was, at several periods of its history in alternate succession, observed to become pestilential or salubrious, as these public works were suffered to fall into decay, or were repaired and renewed.

The different opinions of the origin of Yellow Fever, offer us only the alternative of a more rigid quarantine, or of more vigorous internal measures. Every step of increasing restriction in our system of quarantine, has only served to shew more clearly the domestic origin of the disease. If an entire prohibition of West-India trade, or a prohibition during the summer and autumn, were imposed by law, the effect would soon be sufficient to banish every doubt from the mind of the public. How far the advantage of unanimous conviction might be supposed to countervail the burthen of such restrictions for a short period of years, I shall not undertake to decide.

But whatever opinion may be embraced, the present moment is certainly not the time for the indulgence of apathy or inactivity. If the legislature, in their wisdom, should still think that this disease is introduced from abroad, they are bound by the strongest obligations to extend the powers of quarantine, by additional restrictions. The conveniencies of trade are not to be put in competition with the ravages of yellow fever. If it be necessary to resign the freedom of commerce, or to incur the miseries of pestilence, let the former be freely abandoned.

It is likewise my duty, before I conclude, to suggest whatever it may be deemed adviseable to do towards the removal of existing nuisances, and the improvement of the salubrity of the city. This task has been, in some degree, anticipated in my letter to Governor Clinton, after the epidemic in 1803. Unfortunately, some of the requisite measures will demand great expense, and must bring to a test the liberality, enterprize and public spirit of the city and State. Among the improvements of the most urgent and immediate necessity, I consider the following, to wit; *Water*, obtained from a distant source, of pure quality, and in quantity sufficient to allow a constant, plentiful, and increasing expenditure ; *Sewers*, of such number, capacity and construction, as completely to drain all the low and marshy districts, to carry away all filth, and to be constantly washed by a brisk current of water ; a new arrangement and construction of wharves, docks, &c. so as to face the margin of the two rivers with a stone quay, impervious to water ; a prohibition to make a single additional foot of artificial ground on either of the rivers ; a different modification of privies, which are every day becoming more and more an alarming nuisance, and will soon underlay with filth a large portion of the city ; a better plan of paving, more particularly as respects the construction of gutters, &c. ; the draining of all stagnant waters in the town and neighbourhood, the filling up, levelling and paving all low and depressed lots and places of whatever description ; and a prohibition hereafter to inter dead bodies in any part of the city. Many other objects, which would require much minuteness of detail, likewise demand attention ; and will acquire great additional importance from the rapid progress of building and population.

I have the honour to be,
    With great respect,
        Your Excellency's most obedient
        And humble servant,
            EDWARD MILLER,
                Resident Physician.

Appendix.

UNDER this title, it is intended to lay before the reader some proofs and illustrations of the principles delivered in the foregoing Report, which could not properly be admitted into the letter itself, and which are too long to have been conveniently subjoined in the form of Notes.

——◆——

On the analogy, as to localities and diseases, between the cities of Rome and New-York.

IT is from the south of Europe, and chiefly from *Spain* and *Italy*, that inquirers into the endemic diseases of the United States may expect to derive the most valuable lessons of time and experience. The writings of the Italian physicians in particular, are full of instruction on this subject; and it is to be lamented, that this instruction has not been more eagerly sought for, and more generally obtained by their American brethren.

By considering the following account of the localities and diseases of *Rome*, given by BAGLIVI, and comparing them with those of *New-York*, we perceive how exactly like causes will produce like effects, in the old and in the new continent.

" Ut res exemplo fiat clarior, exponemus breviter,
" quæ nos Romæ circa aëris temperiem, & medendi me-
" thodum quotidiano usu experimur. Aër Romanus
" septem collibus, Orbis dominis, hodie interclusus, na-
" turâ humidus est & gravis; experimento namque con-
" stat, quod si quis paulo longius a frequentia tectorum
" processerit, quantam cœli gravitatem atque intempe-
" riem manifesto concipiet. Insaluberrimis Austri, Africi
" atque Euronoti flatibus obnoxius: ab æstivis caloribus
" interdum tantopere exardescit, ut mirum non videatur,

" si Consulibus L. Valerio Potito, & M. Manlio, Pesti-
" lentia orta sit in agro Romano, *ob siccitates & nimios*
" *solis calores*, teste Livio, lib. V. His aliisque de causis
" infra dicendis, Incolæ urbis temperamento præditi sunt
" melancholico, subfusco, & nonnulli subpallido cutis
" colore, habitu corporis macilento potius quam pingui ;
" levi de causa capite afficiuntur, & iis morbis potissimum
" subjacent, quos aëris gravitas solct producere, sicuti
" sunt pulmonis vitia, febres malignæ, cachexiæ, pallores
" vultus, incubus, tabes & consimiles. Porro aër Roma-
" nus squallidus quoque est & insalubris, non quidem
" omnibus in locis, sed iis potissimum, quæ deficientibus
" ædificiis, pigro atque immoto aëre sordescunt ; muito
" magis si Tiberi adhærent, vel convallium instar, mon-
" tibus obsepiuntur, aut exhalationibus subjacent quas
" veteres parietinæ, cryptæ, & antiquorum ædificiorum
" rudera emittunt. Ex quo patet Regionem Circi Max-
" imi, inter Palatinum atque Aventinum sitam, omnemque
" illum campum qui inter Aventinum, ac Tiberim, por-
" tamque Ostiensem, jacet, plane noxium esse & damna-
" bilem. Sed ut rem universim definiam. Quæcunque
" loca crebris ædificiis ambiuntur, atque editiora sunt, in
" septentrionem atque orientem spectant, & multum a
" Tiberi distant, salubriora : Contra, quæ sejuncta sunt,
" & remota a frequentibus tectis, situque sunt humili, ac
" maxime in convallibus, tum propiora Tiberi, in meri-
" diem atque occasum spectantia, minus salubriora judi-
" cantur : Quibus etiam in locis (quod sane mirum)
" brevissimi intervalli discrimine, hic aliquantum salubris
" existimatur aër ; illic contra noxius & damnabilis.

    " Insalubritatem hanc urbani aëris, fovet magna ex
" parte adjacens Latium ; quod undequaque coronâ mon-
" tium circumcingitur, excepto tractu illo, quâ mediter-
" raneum vergit, ubi in planitiem desinit. Vetus enim
" Latium desertum feré hodie est & squallidum ; Austri
" flatibus immediatè objicitur ; & variis ejusdem in locis,

" insaluberrimus aër observatur, utpotè circa Ostiam &
" Portum, æstivo præsertim tempore ; quo quidem si
" aliquis in præfatis aliisque Latii locis pernoctaverit, &
" exinde urbem revertatur, corripitur statim maligna
" febri, quam vulgo, ex mutatione aëris dicunt ; estque
" febris hæc sui generis, ab aliis febribus, alias agnoscen-
" tibus causas summopere differens, tum in methodo cu-
" rativa, tum in symptomatis eandem concomitantibus."

Georg. Baglivi Oper. Omn. pag. 157, 158.

LANCISI, in his valuable work *De Noxiis Paludum Efflu-viis*, confirms the facts stated by BAGLIVI, and adds many others which are extremely important. In his account of a malignant epidemic, in the summer and autumn of 1695, which ravaged a particular district of the city of Rome to such a degree as nearly to depopulate it, he traces the dis-ease to its cause in the following words :

" Nemo sane luctuosa funera per id temporis Romæ con-
" spiciens, fœtoremque in vicis illis persentiens, dubius
" hæsit, quin causa malignarum, perniciosarumque febrium,
" quæ publice vagabantur, fuerit multitudo stagnantium et
" corruptarum aquarum, tum in scrobibus pratorum, tum
" in magna cloaca, atque in fossa potissimum Hadrianæ ar-
" cis. Tellus jam erat humida, cum Tiberis propter mag-
" nam vim aquæ bis auctus est ; atque idcirco non solum
" scrobes, ac fossæ pratorum et Arcis exhauriri non potue-
" runt ; verum quod maxime aëris insalubritatem inducit,
" sordes, quæ pluviis prolutæ everruntur, ac dilabuntur, iis
" in canalibus atque in cloacis subsistere coactæ sunt. Si-
" mul etiam per humiliora Leoninæ civitatis loca exunda-
" vit, subterraneasque cellas, multosque pauperum puteos
" hic illic contemeravit. Posthæc, negligentia eorum, qui
" rebus publicis, atque eidem præsertim Arci præerant, nul-
" lum studium purgandis hisce regionibus adhibitum fuit.
" Hinc mira hæc proluvies in limosam paludem sensim in-
" tra fossas scrobesque conversa, virescere, jam urgente

" æstu, fermentari, computrescere, variaque insecta admit-
" tere cœpit. His vero malis accessit etiam frequens affla
" tus Vulturni, austrinorumque ventorum, qui a medio
" Maio usque ad Septembrem identidem recurrentes, non
" tantum deteriori putredini immotarum aquarum, verum
" faciliori quoque sublimationi ac delationi malignorum
" effluviorum non in vicinas duntaxat ædes, sed etiam
" usque ad finitimas adversasque regiones, ansam præbue-
" runt."

Lancis. Oper. Var. Tom. 1. *p.* 189.

On the antiquity of the Yellow Fever.

IT has been contended by some, that the yellow fever
is a modern disease, and utterly unknown to Europe,
except when imported there from America. A slight inspection of the writings of HIPPOCRATES, who flourished
upwards of four hundred years before the Christian æra,
will be sufficient to prove that he was familiarly acquainted with it, and had observed it under its most malignant
and fatal forms.

The two symptoms which are considered as most characteristic of this fever, are *yellowness of skin*, and *black
vomiting*. A great number of passages might be adduced
to shew that Hippocrates frequently met with these symptoms in the malignant fevers which fell under his care.
I shall mention only such as are clear, pointed, and incapable of being mistaken.   In the ninth section of his book
of Crises, he lays it down as a maxim, that " *in burning
fevers, a yellowness of skin appearing on the fifth day, and
accompanied by hiccough, is a fatal symptom.*"*   This is a

---

* *For the sake of removing all doubt on this subject, it
is proper to submit the original to the reader's consideration :—*

Ἐν τοισι καυσοισιν ἐαν ἐπιγενηται ἰκτερος και λυξη πεμπταιω
ἐοντι, θανατωδες ὑποςροφαι λαμβανονται.

very brief, exact, and appropriate description of the disease. A greater number are said to die of yellow fever on the sixth than any other day of the disease ; and it very frequently happens that appearances of yellowness are discovered on the fifth, which, at that period, and accompanied by hiccough, constitute a fatal symptom. When the description which Hippocrates gives of *Causus*, or *Burning Fever*, is duly recollected, and there is connected with this fever the occurrence of yellow skin, accompanied with hiccough, on the fifth day ; a character results, which can apply to no other disease in the world but yellow fever. And it would be exceedingly difficult, in so few words, to present a more expressive delineation of that distemper.

The terrible symptom of *black vomiting* is also frequently mentioned by Hippocrates, and represented as being of fatal import. He uses the phrases μελαινα χολη black bile, μελανα εμετον black vomit, and μελανων εμετον the vomiting of black matter. In the twelfth section of his Prognostics, he asserts, that if the matter vomited be of a livid or black colour, it betokens ill. In the first section of the first book of his *Coan Prognostics*, he enumerates black vomiting in a catalogue of the most fatal symptoms. And also in the fourth section of the same book, he considers porraceous, livid or black vomiting as indications of great malignancy.*

The importance of this conclusion is further illustrated and confirmed by adverting to the well known fact, that Hippocrates practised physic for a considerable portion of his life, in parts of Greece situated nearly in the same parallel of latitude with those in the United States, where the yellow fever has produced its greatest ravages.

See *Medical Repository, Hex. II. Vol.* 3, *page* 107.

---

* Ει δε ειη το εμευμενον πρασοειδες, η πελιον, η μελαν, οτι αν η τουτεων των χρωματων, νομιζειν χρη πονηρον ειται.

On another account, the writings of Hippocrates offer important instruction concerning malignant fevers. Not the least reference to *contagion* is to be found in any part of them. If personal intercourse between the sick and the well had been the means of spreading these fevers from one individual or from one family to another, it is incredible that so prominent and glaring a fact should have escaped the notice of a person endowed with such talents for extensive, accurate and discriminating observation.

Yellow Fever indigenous in the Island of Minorca.

BY the following quotation from *Cleghorn's Observations on the Epidemical Diseases of Minorca, from the year* 1744 *to* 1749, page 175 & 176, it appears that yellow fever often prevailed in that island more than sixty years ago, and that it was by no means considered as a new or extraordinary disease. It also appears, that the characteristic symptoms of yellow fever are often superinduced on the intermittent fevers of that place, and that their common tertian fevers are only a lower grade of yellow fever. The island of Minorca is situated nearly in our latitude.

" But the utmost danger is to be apprehended, if a few
" drops of blood fall from the nose : if black matter like
" the grounds of coffee, is discharged upwards or down-
" wards : if the urine is of a dark hue and a strong offen-
" sive smell : if the whole skin is tinged with a deep yel-
" low, or any where discoloured with livid spots or suffu-
" sions : if a cadaverous smell is perceptible about the
" patient's bed : if in the time of the fit he continues cold
" and chilly, without being able to recover heat ; or if he
" becomes extremely hot, speechless and stupid ; has
" frequent sighs, groans, or hiccoughs ; and lies constantly
" on his back, with a ghastly countenance, his eyes half
" shut, his mouth open, his belly swelled to an enormous

L

" size, with an obstinate costiveness, or an involuntary
" discharge of the excrements : which formidable symp-
" toms, as they seldom appear before the third revolution
" of the disease, so they frequently come on, both in
" double and simple intermittents, during the fourth,
" fifth, or sixth period, even where the smallest danger
" was not foreseen." The author likewise adds, in a note,
that " The English in Minorca are more liable than the na-
" tives to become yellow in these fevers."

On Yellow Fever in the interior of the Country.

SPORADIC cases of this disease are occasionally observed in all parts of the country. They are found more frequently and in greater number in low and marshy districts,
near lakes, mill-ponds, swamps, &c. The most respecta-
ble physicians in the country so universally concur in this
observation, that it would be unreasonable to contest the
fact.

In some of the more exposed situations, and after very
hot and damp summers, the yellow fever often assumes an
epidemic appearance in the country. The malignant disease at Catskill in this State, in the year 1803, (see *Medical Repository*, vol. 8, page 105) affords an instance of this
kind. In the year 1793, it prevailed in many parts of the
country in the eastern, middle and southern States, where
no suspicion of contagion could exist.

DR. ANTHON, of this city, whose accurate acquaintance
with the pestilential epidemics of New-York enables him to
decide in the most satisfactory manner, assures me he has
often seen the same disease in the interior country, and
particularly in the low situations near the river *Illinois*, after an extensive inundation of that river, succeeded by hot
weather.

MR. VOLNEY found yellow fever in several parts of the
interior western country, during his travels in America, and

describes the disease with so much accuracy and force, that no doubt of his testimony can be entertained.
See his View of the Climate and Soil of the United States.

Out of a great mass of particular instances of the appearances of yellow fever in situations inaccessible to foreign contagion, I shall only now select the following :

Extract from Mr. Andrew Ellicott's Voyage down the River Ohio, in the month of November, 1796.

" *November* 15*th.*

" Arrived at Galliopolis about 11 o'clock in the morning.—This village is a few miles below the mouth of the Great Kanhaway, on the west side of the Ohio river, and situated on a high bank ; it is inhabited by a number of miserable French families. Many of the inhabitants, this season, fell victims to the yellow fever. The mortal cases were generally attended with the black vomiting. This disorder certainly originated in the town, and, in all probability, from the filthiness of the inhabitants, added to an unusual quantity of animal and vegetable putrefaction in a number of small ponds and marshes within the village.

" The fever could not have been taken there from the Atlantic States, as my boat was the first that descended the river after the fall of the waters in the spring : neither could it have been taken from New-Orleans, as there is no communication, at that season of the year, up the river, from the latter to the former of those places : moreover, the distance is so great, that a boat would not have time to ascend the river, after the disorder appeared that year in New-Orleans, before the winter would set in."

See Ellicott's Journal.

The following fact is communicated by Dr. Watkins, from his personal knowledge.

There is a village called *New-Design*, about fifteen miles from the Mississippi, and twenty miles from St. Louis, containing about forty houses and two hundred souls. It is on high ground, but surrounded by ponds. In 1797, the yellow fever carried off fifty-seven of the inhabitants, or more than a fourth. No person had arrived at that village from any part of the country where this fever had prevailed, for more than twelve months preceding. Our informant resided in the village at the time ; and, having seen the disease in Philadelphia, he declares it to be the same that prevailed at New-Design. He also mentions an Indian village depopulated by the same disease two or three years before.

See Medical Repository, vol. 4, *page* 74.

Fever, with black vomiting, in the middle part of Pennsylvania, west of the Susquehannah.

" The fever which prevailed, in the autumn and winter of 1799, in Nittany and Bald-Eagle Valley, in Mifflin county, Pennsylvania, proved, in a number of cases, mortal. Bald-Eagle Valley, situated about 200 miles N. N. W. of Philadelphia, is low, abounding with much stagnated water in ponds, which, from the dryness of the season, became very putrid and offensive to the smell. Near to these waters the fever prevailed with great malignity. It was ushered in by chills, with pains in the back, limbs and head, which, in 48 or 60 hours, carried off the patients.— They discharged vast quantities of filth from the stomach, of the consistence and appearance of coffee-grounds, so offensive in smell as to produce nausea, and even vomiting, in the attendants. The fæces also had the same appear-ance. In many the disease terminated by profuse discharges of blood from the anus and vagina.

Ibid. page 75.

On DR. CHISHOLM's *singular opinions concerning Yellow Fever.*

IT is well known that this gentleman contends for the production of a *new* and *peculiar pestilential disease,* which he supposes to have been imported by the *ship Hankey,* in the year 1793, from Boullam, on the coast of Africa.* He believes this new distemper to have been spread through the W.India islsnds and transmitted to this country. He admits that the yellow fever of the West-Indies, is not a contagious disease. The importers and contagionists in the United States, assuming his opinion, and fortifying themselves by his authority, assert that our epidemics are not the yellow fever of the West-Indies, but a continuation of the new and peculiar Boullam fever.

But the slightest examination of the subject is sufficient to satisfy an impartial inquirer, that the Boullam fever of Dr. Chisholm and the yellow fever of the West-Indies, are precisely the same disease ; and that only such occasional variations of grade have been observed in it, as are found in the different epidemic seasons of all pestilential distempers. The ravages of pestilence in the West-Indies, since the pretended introduction of the Boullam disease, among a given number of Europeans or other strangers recently arrived, or among the natives themselves, are not greater than they were fifty years ago, or during the war of the American Revolution. The great body of physicians and people in the West-Indies, do not find the fever now prevailing at all different from what it was many years before the arrival of the ship Hankey from Boullam. The descriptions of the disease by physicians who wrote forty, fifty and sixty years ago, precisely agree with what is now observed in those islands and on this continent. And in this city, the yellow fever prevailed in the autumn of 1791, two years before the supposed arrival of the Boullam disease by the ship Hankey.

Without recurring, however, to facts of this kind, Dr. Chisholm's doctrine, considered in itself, cannot stand the test of examination. All his leading assertions concerning the pretended introduction of the Boullam fever into the West-Indies, are positively denied by Mr. Paiba,

*An Essay on the Malignant Pestilential Fever, &c. 2d Edit. in 2 vols.

a gentleman of intelligence and unblemished character, who was on board of the ship charged with the importation, during the whole of the voyage. The narrative itself of the voyage, and of the disease supposed to have been imported, betrays inherent evidence of mistake. And even if Dr. Chisholm's story be admitted, it is only an instance of malignant disease generated in a vessel, as he does not pretend to derive it from the Africans.

Dr. Chisholm makes a very elaborate attempt to discriminate the features of the Boullam fever from those of the yellow fever of the West-Indies. It is apparent that there is no foundation for the distinction ; and that he only describes different grades of the same disease, modified and rendered more malignant at one time than another, by peculiarities of season. This happens with respect to all epidemic diseases. The measles, for example, in one season, are *mild and safe*, at another, they are *malignant and fatal ;* in one epidemic they are *highly inflammatory*, in another they may be *highly putrid;* yet are they not essentially the same disease? But, admitting, for argument's sake, the distinction contended for by Dr. C. it may be still asserted that, in his description of the ordinary yellow fever of the West-Indies, and not in that of the Boullam fever, he gives the character of the disease which has so often prevailed in this city.

It is creditable to the candour of Dr. Chisholm that he seems lately, in a considerable degree, at least in effect, to have given up his favourite opinion. He now admits that a disease, similar to that of Boullam, has been since generated on board of a filthy ship from England. It is proper to give his own words, as expressed in an extract of a letter to Dr. Davidson, dated Demarara, August 10, 1800, a period of seven years after the formation of his first opinion.

" A fever of a most alarming nature has most fatally prevailed since the beginning of July. I have visited a few of the sick at the request of Doctors Dunkin and

Lloyd in town, and of Dr. Ord on this coast ; and ⨪ have no hesitation in pronouncing it a fever of infection. Its features are, almost without exception, precisely those of the malignant pestilential fever of Grenada of 1793 and 1794. It is fully as fatal, as rapid, and as insidious. Its origin, as far as it has been ascertained by the gentlemen I have mentioned, seems to be similar. A ship arrived about the beginning of July or end of June from Liverpool, after touching at Surinam. The filth on board, occasioned by a cargo of horses, and the extreme neglect of the officers and crew, was such as beggars description."

See Medical Repository, vol. 5, page 229.

Thefe facts, thus presented by Dr. Chisholm himself, form a luminous and instructive commentary on his former opinion, which he had published with great confidence, and which has been implicitly adopted and acted on by the contagionists in the United States. In 1793, he pronounced the malignant disease of Grenada, which, as was observed before, he believed to have been imported from the coast of Africa, a " *nova pestis*," a peculiar, original, foreign pestilence, recently generated and utterly unknown before, endued with a new and distinct character, possessing new powers of devastation, and capable of propagating itself by contagion throughout the world. As he considered it to have been engendered on board of the Hankey, in consequence of the accumulation of filth, the crowding of a great number of persons within a small space, and the heat of the atmosphere in which the vessel was immersed ; he must have ascribed whatever peculiarity he supposed it to possess, to the peculiar state of the air on the coast of Africa ; for he did not pretend to derive it originally from the inhabitants of Africa, or any modification of contagion. No other circumstance of the case, therefore, except some unknown singularity of the African atmosphere, could occasion this alleged instance of the generation of pestilence in a ship to differ from other cases in which malignant fevers are produced in filthy, crowded and unventilated vessels, in hot climates or during hot seasons. But in the year 1800, while the flames of the Boullam disease lighted up in 1793, were still raging far and wide, and destroying the people of the West-Indies and of the American continent, he finds another *"nova pestis,"* generated in a ship from England, which had touched at Surinam, and had become very filthy from a cargo of horses ; and what is wonderful, he finds this pestilence, thus originating in a ship from England, possessing *features, almost without exception, precisely those of the malignant, pestilensial fever of Grenada, of 1793 and 1794 ; fully as fatal, as rapid, and as insidious.*—It appears then that the facts advanced by Dr. C. in the latter case (even admitting those concerning the Hankey to be true) instead of supporting his doctrine of *novelty and peculiarity in the fever of Boullam,* go too far for his purpose, and establish the general principle, that filthy, crowded, and unventilated vessels, immersed in a certain degree of heat and dampness, may generate malignant fever in all parts of the world where such circumstances are found,—which is precisely the principle for which the advocates of local and domestic origin have always contended.

As to Dr. C's opinion of the contagiousness of these fevers, it rests upon the same vague and delusive foundation with the popular, or rather vulgar inference of contagion, in all cases where a disease attacks a great number of persons in the same vicinity ; which has been sufficiently refuted in a former part of this Report.

𝕽eport

OF

THE GENERAL COMMITTEE

OF

HEALTH.

M

THE COMMITTEE OF THE BOARD OF HEALTH, APPOINTED
TO CONSIDER WHAT PREVENTIVE MEASURES MAY BE
NECESSARY TO SECURE THE HEALTH OF THE CITY OF
NEW-YORK,

—REPORT—

THAT the introduction of a copious supply of pure and
wholesome water as well for domestic use, as for the purpose of sprinkling the streets and cleansing the kennels, during the summer season, is essentially necessary. As water constitutes a large proportion of the liquids we take, and
is constantly used in the processes of cooking, it is scarcely
necessary to prove that it ought to be pure. As it is the
basis of all ablution, and the principle means of cleanliness,
whether as to domestic or public nuisances, it ought to be
plentiful as well as pure. The experience of all old and
large cities proves, that water procured from any source
within their limits, or in their neighbourhood, is impure
and unwholesome; and that it always becomes necessary
to obtain it from some distant place, beyond the reach of
contamination from the city, and in quantity, copious, steady
and inexhaustible. All schemes therefore, for procuring
potable and culinary water from any source within the city,
or in the neighbourhood, ought to be rejected, and some
arrangement devised as soon as possible, at whatever expence, to bring it in sufficient quantity, and of the greatest
purity, from some river or stream, that rises at a distance.
Our sister city of Philadelphia has set us an example of a
noble and costly establishment for this object. On this
point they are greatly in advance of us. There is reason
to believe, that they are already reaping the fruits of this
provident and wise plan. The yellow fever of the last season, though it appeared sporadically all over that city,

was only epidemic in those districts to which the advantages of a copious supply of pure water, sufficient to scour gutters and wash streets, had not extended.

That common sewers ought to be constructed in such streets of this city as are of sufficient descent to the river, in order to drain cellars and low grounds, and to discharge kitchen and backwater under ground as much as possible. It is one of the first and most essential objects, in a system intended to improve the healthiness of the city, to devise some adequate plan for *draining* all the low, moist and marshy grounds. It is conceived, that nothing can produce any great or permanent good effect, without this improvement. Whether this draining can be best accomplished by sewers, by canals, or by any other means, is a question which can only be determined by a skilful intelligent engineer.

That the line of wharves along our shores ought to be faced with solid stone masonry, constructed in such manner as to be impervious to water. To face the margin of the East and North Rivers, on a permanent line, with stone, and to render this line impervious to water, seems also to be a measure of the first necessity, towards recovering the healthiness of the city. While the present construction of wharves and docks is suffered to remain, not only the filth, which finds admittance and settles among the logs and stones, must be very pernicious ; but the water, which is incessantly transuding, keeps in a state of moisture, and consequently in the worst state to be operated upon by heat, all the animal and vegetable offals, which overspreads and forms so large a proportion of the *made ground*. While water is allowed to pass in this constant and copious manner from the rivers, it is impossible that the made ground should ever be dry, consolidated or wholesome. Whatever of a decaying and corrupting quality is to be found in it, by the aid of this water, when acted upon by the high heat of summer, will be prepared to emit the most virulent miasmata, and particularly that daily and hourly succession of them, which no breeze, nor even hurricane could effectually sweep away. If this line of stone work were properly constructed, there is reason to believe that all the cellars in the lower parts of the town (especially if the aid of sewers were likewise introduced) would be rendered safe, wholesome, and applicable to any of the useful purposes for which they are designed. And it may, perhaps, deserve consideration, how far the preservation of these cellars for their present purposes, and the eventual saving to be expected from a permanent erection of stone, instead of the temporary erection of wood, subject to continual decay and dilapidation, and requiring to be rebuilt at short intervals, aided by a reasonable augmentation of the present rates of wharfage, would go towards reimbursing the great expence of this improvement.

That the interment of dead bodies within the city ought to be prohibited. A vast mass of decaying animal matter, produced by the superstition of interring dead bodies near to churches, and which has been accumulating for a long lapse of time, is now deposited in many of the most populous parts of the city. It is impossible that such a quantity of these animal remains, even if placed at the greatest depth of interment commonly practised, should continue to be inoffensive and safe. It is difficult, if not impracticable, to determine to what distance around, the matter extricated during the process of putrefaction may spread ; and by pervading the ground, tainting the waters, and perhaps emitting noxious exhalations into the atmosphere, do great mischief. But if it should be decided still to persist in the practice of interment within the city, it ought to be judged necessary to order the envelopement of the bodies in some species of calcareous earth, either quick lime or chalk. The present burial grounds might serve extremely well for plantations of grove and forest trees, and thereby, instead of remaining receptacles of putrefying matter and hot beds of miasmata, might be rendered useful and ornamental to the city. This growing evil must be corrected at some period ; for it is encreasing and extending by daily aggregation to a mass already very large, and the sooner it is arrested, the less violence will be done to the feelings and habits of our fellow citizens.

That the planting of trees and other healthy vegetables ought to be encouraged. There is good reason to believe, that frequent extensive and numerous plantations of trees, and cultivating with care, wherever room can be found, the smaller plants, would be an important step towards rendering the city more like the country, as to the condition of its atmosphere, and thereby diminishing the prevalenee of pestilential diseases. It is believed, that ten or twenty times, or perhaps a greater proportion of vegetable growth, beyond the existing amount, might be introduced into this city, not only without inconvenience or injury to the but public so as greatly to conduce to its pleasantness, ornament, healthfulness, and the protection of its inhabitants from the effects of the direct rays of the sun in summer and in the beginning of autumn.

That a scientific and skilful engineer should be employed to assist in projecting and executing the several objects embraced in this report. It cannot be too frequently inculcated on the minds of our citizens, that in all the improvements to be undertaken in New-York, we ought as far as possible to avail ourselves of the examples exhibited in the old cities of the eastern continent, and to admit only such things as have been sanctioned by the award of time and experience. It is especially proper to direct our researches to the southern parts of Europe, and particularly to Spain and Italy, which lie under corresponding degrees of latitude with many parts of the United States ; but in order to obtain this knowledge in so precise and accurate a manner as to be applicable to our purposes, it will be requisite to consult and to retain in employment some able and enlightened engineer, who has added to the advantages of a regular and scientific edu‑cation, much experimental and practical acquaintance with business, the improvements of travel, and that ma‑turity of character which can only be derived from long reflection and experience. Such a person ought to be ob‑tained, from whatever distance, or at whatever expence, it may be necessary to procure him. It is only by pro‑viding in this manner, that the corporation of this city can hope to escape censure, to erect works and establish im‑provements of solid and lasting utility, such as will do credit to the city and themselves, and such as will endure the test of time and criticism of posterity.

That all cellars subject to the influence of tides or backwater, should be filled up level with the streets, and that all lots should be regulated in such manner as to dis‑charge the water freely into the streets. That no cellars which may be found damp and obnoxious to health, should, on any condition, be inhabited. That all vaults of privies which may be deemed unwholesome, either from being situate in confined places, or from whatever cause, should be filled up, and tubs substituted in their place.

And whereas various houses, in different parts of the city, have on the recurrence of every malignant fever, proved to be the principal seats of disease, and the graves of their tenants, the committee suggest the propriety of prohibiting the same to be let or occupied as dwell‑ing houses, that they be converted into ware-houses, and that any injury sustained by the proprietors be defrayed by the public.

That no further encroachment be made into Hudson river, than what may be absolutely necessary for public

basons and quays ; and that no buildings be erected beyond the present boundary of Washington-street.

That more extensive accommodations ought to be provided at Bellevue Hospital for the reception of sick patients ;
and that a pay hospital be erected for the accommodation
of such persons, whose circumstances may afford the expence.

The committee further recommend the following amend-
ments to the quarantine law : that all vessels arriving from
the West Indies and the Mississippi, during the months of
July, August and September, shall remain at the Quarantine Ground not less than four days after their arrival, and
that no intercourse shall be permitted, during that period,
between the crew or crews of said vessels and the city of
New-York, unless subject to such restrictions as shall be
prescribed by the Health Officer. And that such vessels
shall, moreover, be detained at the Quarantine Ground for
a longer term than the aforesaid four days, if, in the opinion
of the Health Officer, such detention may appear necessary.

All which is respectfully submitted.

    (Signed)

        WYNANT VAN ZANT, Jr.
        EDWARD MILLER,
        JOHN PINTARD.

New-York, Jan. 20, 1806.

ENUMERATION OF THE INHABITANTS

OF THE

CITY OF NEW-YORK.

———•◦•———

To the Honourable the Mayor, Aldermen and Commonalty
of the City of New-York,

THE City Inspector has the honour to report, that in conformity with the order of the Common Council, an enumeration has been taken of the jurors in the city and county of New-York, agreeably to " An act of the Legislature regulating trials of issues, and for returning able and sufficient jurors," passed 31st March, 1801, which enumeration also comprehends the number of inhabitants who retired from the city, during the prevalence of the malignant fever in 1805, together with the total population.

Which is respectfully submitted.

JOHN PINTARD.

WARDS.	White Inhabitants.		People of Colour and Free Negroes.		Slaves.		TOTAL.	Persons who retired from the city during the malignant fever in 1805.
	Males.	Females.	Males.	Females.	Males.	Females		
FIRST...........	3,422	3,748	37	37	186	249	7,679	6,112
SECOND.........	3,414	3,653	72	101	118	182	7,550	5,961
THIRD...........	3,283	3,597	106	119	104	162	7,371	4,152
FOURTH.........	4,346	4,520	70	87	68	143	9,234	4,320
FIFTH	5,320	3,993	358	438	85	146	12,340	3,452
SIXTH...........	4,101	4,266	183	253	59	99	8,961	224
SEVENTH	8,053	7,498			38	79	15,668	2,775
EIGHTH.........	2,420	2,134	38	61	49	70	4,772	
NINTH............	1,025	959			111	100	2,195	
	65,384	36,578	864	1,096	818	1,230	75,770	26,996

Extract from the original returns on file in this office.

JOHN PINTARD, *City Inspector*.

City Inspector's Office,
February 24th, 1806.

According to the Census taken by order of Congress in 1801, the population of this City amounted to

Free White Males - - - - -	26,727
Do. do. Females - - - - -	27,394
Other Free Persons - - - - -	3,499
Slaves - - - - - - - -	2,869
	60,489
Increase of population in 5 years, at the rate of 25 per cent. }	15,281
	75,770

The total number of Cases of Malignant Fever, which occurred in the City of New-York in 1805, was - - - - - - - - - - - - -   645

The Deaths by the same disease, in the City, at Bellevue and the Marine Hospital, amounted to   302

viz.

WARDS.	Cases of Malig-nant Fever.	Deaths.
FIRST - - - - - - - -	105	37
SECOND - - - - - - - -	93	45
THIRD - - - - - - - -	67	28
FOURTH - - - - - - - -	79	33
FIFTH - - - - - - - -	90	25
SIXTH - - - - - - - -	83	18
SEVENTH - - - - - - -	101	25
EIGHTH - - - - - - - -	26	9
NINTH - - - - - - - -	2	2
BELLEVUE - - - - - -		52
MARINE HOSPITAL - -		28
	645	302

Statistical.—By the Enumeration of the In-habitants of this city recently publifhed, the progrefs of population for the laft 5 years appears to be at the rate of 25 per cent. Should our city continue to increafe in the fame proportion during the prefent century, the agregate number. at its clofe, will far exceed that of any other city in the old woild, Pekin not except-ed : as will appear from the following table.

Progrefs of Population in the city of New-York computed at the rate of 25 per cent every 5 years

1805	75,770
1810	94.715
1815	110,390
1820	147 987
1825	184,9 3
1830	231,228
1835	289,035
1840	361,293
1845	451,616
1850	564,520
1855	705 650
1860	882,062
1865	1,10 ,577
1870	1,378,221
1875	1,722,776
1880	2,153,470
1885	2,69 ,837

1890	3,364,796
1895	4,205,995
1900	5 257,493

From this table it appears, that the population of this city, fixty years hence, will confiderably exceed the reputed population of the cities of Paris and London. Cities and nations, however, like individuals, experience their rife, progrefs, and decline It is hardly probable that New-York will be fo highly favoured as to prove an exception. Wars, peftilence, and political convulfions, muft be our lot, and be taken into calculation. With every allowance, however, for the " numerous ills which life is heir to," from our advantageous maritime fituation, and the increafe of agriculture and commerce, our numbers will in all probability, at the end of this century, exceed thofe of any other city in the world, Pekin alone excepted.

From the data here furnifhed, the politician, financier, and above all the fpeculator in townlots, (a fubject, to our fhame be it fpoken, which abforbs every generous paffion) may draw various and interefting inferences.